The Heart Attack Prevention & Recovery Handbook

The Heart Attack Prevention & Recovery Handbook

by

Jack Gillis, M.D.

Hartley & Marks
PUBLISHERS

Published by Hartley & Marks, Publishers, Inc.
Box 147 3661 West Broadway
Point Roberts, WA Vancouver, BC
98281 V6R 2B8

Library of Congress Cataloging-in-Publication Data

Gillis, Jack, 1925 –
The heart attack prevention & recovery handbook / by Jack Gillis.
p. cm.
Includes bibliographical references and index.
ISBN 0-88179-118-0
1. Coronary heart disease—Popular works. I. Title. II. Title: Heart attack prevention and recovery.

RC685.C6G48 1993
616.1'23025—dc20 –93–1 6946

If not available at your local bookstore, this book may be ordered directly from the publisher. Send the cover price plus three dollars fifty for shipping costs to the above address.

Contents

Acknowledgments

I am grateful to many for their influence, cooperation, and help in writing this book. The notion and impetus came from the people I serve: patients. I am grateful to the physicians who have allowed me to cooperate in the care of their patients, and to the far-flung researchers whose scientific studies are the back-bone of the book.

Thanks to my wife Marion, for her unfailing support. In my office, Dorothy Dodd, Carol McBryde, and Karen Armitage have been of particular help with suggestions. My thanks to daughters Susan, Sheelagh, Pamela, and Mary for their encouragement and helpful suggestions. I am grateful, as well, for the professional editorial assistance of Nancy Flight and Claudette Reed-Upton, and for the efficient and courteous service of the British Columbia Medical Library Service.

The end product of this enterprise is like a sculpture with many shavings left on the floor. I am very indebted to the perspicacity and direction provided by the editorial staff of Hartley & Marks Publishers, especially Sue Tauber, but also Elizabeth McLean. From them I have learned a lot.

Introduction

This book will give you the basic, practical information you need to know to keep your heart healthy. It offers clear, easy-to-understand guidelines based on our most up-to-date knowledge about heart attack prevention.

WHO SHOULD READ THIS BOOK?

This book is for you if:

- *You have been told that your blood cholesterol or triglyceride levels are out of the safe range for your age and gender.* *(See Important, p. xi.)*
- *You are a cigarette smoker.*
- *Your blood pressure is higher than normal.*
- *You have diabetes.*
- *You have had a heart attack.*
- *You have had a coronary artery bypass or coronary angioplasty.*
- *You have angina (angina pectoris)—that is, chest pains, discomfort, or pressure due to insufficient blood flow to the heart muscle.*
- *Your exercise stress test shows early signs that you are at increased risk for a heart attack.*
- *You have a blood relative with premature (before age 55) heart trouble as a result of coronary artery disease (including those who have had coronary artery bypass or angioplasty).*

- *You have a blood relative with too high total cholesterol, or too low HDL cholesterol levels.*
- *You have a partner or spouse or another family member who is at risk for heart attacks.*
- *You want an up-to-date summary of how to significantly reduce your heart attack risk.*

HOW WILL THIS BOOK HELP YOU?

- *This book contains clear, concise information about the risk factors for heart disease, who is at risk, and how to find out if you are at risk.*
- *It also gives step-by-step guidelines for controlling your risk factors.*
- *A chapter on a preventive program tells you what you can do every day to keep your heart healthy.*
- *Other chapters tell you what to do if you are over 60, if you are a woman, or if you have already had a heart attack.*
- *The Progress Chart in Chapter 11 provides a method for you to keep track of your own heart attack risk factors over a period of years. It helps you to work with your doctor to control these risk factors.*
- *There are guidelines showing how your family members can help.*
- *There is a chapter describing the medications that your doctor may prescribe for controlling your high blood pressure or out-of-range blood cholesterol or triglycerides.*
- *Important new research underlying the strategies in the book is summarized in Chapter 14.*
- *The APPENDICES give the fat content and saturated fat content of common foods; food sources and recommended daily supplements of vitamins and minerals; and other useful tables.*
- *The GLOSSARY defines medical terms used in the book.*
- *There is a list of SUGGESTED READING for additional information.*

■ HOW CAN YOU USE THIS BOOK?

- *Use this book to identify the strategies you need to follow to change your lifestyle and lead a longer, healthier, happier life.*
- *Carry it with you as a daily guide for preventive health.*
- *Use the Progress Chart for years to control your risk factors over the long term, and make new goals for yourself.*

Important:
Remember that you *can* enhance your health if you really want to, and by learning how to do it. The light of knowledge opens paths for you.

While nutrition and exercise are cornerstones of prevention, modern medicine continues to find new ways for you to live longer and fruitfully.

If you have extra risk factors for a heart attack be sure to develop your personalized preventive strategies with a doctor properly schooled in this field of medicine.

WHAT IS...*

Atherosclerosis (artery disease)?

A degenerative disease of the arteries. The most common effect is a build-up of cholesterol deposits (plaque), which restricts blood flow. Can also cause an aneurysm (bulging of the artery).

Plaque?

Degenerative built-up "patches" on an artery's inner wall, composed mainly of cholesterol deposits, fibrous tissue, and overgrowth of muscle tissue. The inner layer is called the "fibrous cap." Heart attacks result when this covering becomes fissured and inflamed, permitting an unwanted clot (thrombosis) to occur.

Angina?

Pain or discomfort, usually in the chest, caused by insufficient blood flow to the heart. If it persists for over 20 minutes, it can be a symptom of a heart attack.

Coronary thrombosis?

Sudden and complete closure of a coronary artery, caused by a blood clot in an artery narrowed by atherosclerosis.

Heart attack?

A sudden heart disturbance, sometimes life-threatening, and usually caused by coronary thrombosis.

Myocardial infarct (or infarction)?

The medical term for a heart attack. The death of part of the heart muscle due to a coronary thrombosis stopping the blood flow.

* See also GLOSSARY and INDEX

Are You at Risk for a Heart Attack?

I

■ FACTS ABOUT HEART DISEASE

- *Heart disease kills or disables more adults in industrialized countries than any other disease.*
- *Cancer causes significantly fewer deaths than heart disease.*
- *Each year more than eight out of every 1,000 people in North America between the ages of 35 and 75 die from heart-related causes, the majority from heart attacks.*
- *If you are a man between the ages of 35 and 44, your risk of death from heart disease is relatively low: 46 out of a population of 100,000 die per year. But for many, the groundwork is being laid for trouble a few years later. Between the ages of 55 and 64, the death rate from heart disease has risen by 1,100 percent, and continues its climb with each passing year.*
- *If you are a woman between the ages of 35 and 44, your risk is very low: only 12.5 out of 100,000 die per year. But women experience a 1,700 percent increase in deaths from heart disease between ages 55 and 64, to 213 out of 100,000 each year. (Figures based on research of the white U.S. population.)*
- *Although your risk of dying from a heart attack increases as you age, the majority of victims of the disease which leads to heart attacks—coronary artery disease—are under 65.*
- *If you are unemployable for health reasons, there is a one in three chance it is due to your heart.*

■ RISK FACTORS FOR HEART ATTACKS

Most adults in the industrialized world carry at least one major risk factor for a heart attack. Many have more than one, and each risk factor multiplies, rather than merely adds to, their heart attack risk.

You are at risk for a heart attack if you have any of the following risk factors:

- *You are a man with a high total cholesterol level—that is, over 200 milligrams per deciliter (200 mg/dL), sometimes written as millimoles per liter (5.17 mmol/L).*
- *You are a man with high LDL (low density lipoprotein) cholesterol—that is, above 130 mg/dL (3.4 mmol/L). (See pp. 21 and 30.)*
- *You are a man or a woman with low HDL (high density lipoprotein) cholesterol—that is, under 45 mg/dL (1.16 mmol/L).*

The heart disease death rate rises by over 1,000% between study groups aged 35 to 44, and 55 to 64.

- *Your ratio of total cholesterol to HDL cholesterol is higher than 4.5. (See p. 21.)*
- *You have a high blood trigylceride level—that is, above 204 mg/dL (2.3 mmol/L). (See pp. 22 and 31.)*
- *You have a family history of heart disease.*
- *You have high blood pressure—that is, above 140/90.*
- *You smoke cigarettes.*
- *You do not exercise regularly.*
- *You are a man and over age 45, or a woman and over age 55.*
- *You are overweight.*
- *You are under stress.*
- *You have diabetes.*

In addition to these risk factors, you are also at risk if:

- *You have had a heart attack.*
- *You have recurrent angina (chest pains due to insufficient blood flow to the heart muscle).*
- *You have silent exertional ischemia.*
- *You have had a coronary artery bypass or an angioplasty.*

■ IF YOU HAVE HAD A HEART ATTACK

- *In the United States and Canada, about four of every 1,000 people become victims of a heart attack each year. Half of these people die before reaching the hospital. Of those who make it to hospital, almost two of five die within the next year.*
- *If you have survived a recent heart attack, you may be in a low risk group, or an intermediate, or a high risk group, in respect to your chances of surviving the next few months. Your doctor can use information already on hand to show your prognosis. If you are in an intermediate or high risk group, you will need special attention to protect you. For example, you may require coronary artery bypass or angioplasty (surgery on your coronary arteries) to improve blood flow to the heart.*

Every year, 1 in 250 people in the U.S. and Canada suffers a heart attack.

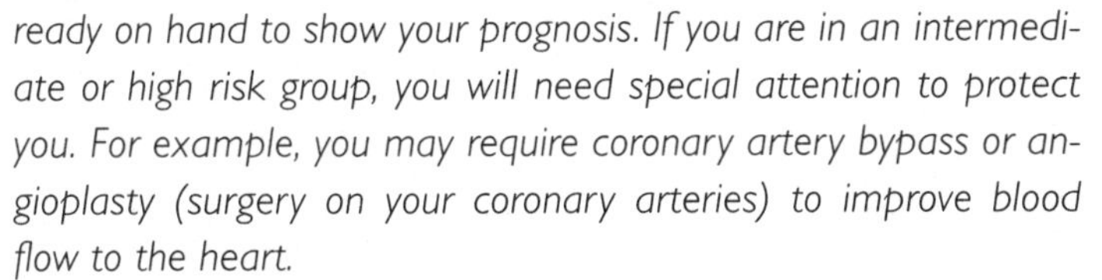

■ IF YOU HAVE CHRONIC, STABLE ANGINA PECTORIS

- *If you have been spared a heart attack but have chronic, stable angina (you can predict when your heart pains will occur), your chances of dying from heart trouble in the next few years are about twice that of your friends of the same age who do not have angina.*
- *Your chances of suffering from a nonfatal heart attack are increased threefold.*

■ IF YOU HAVE HAD A CORONARY ARTERY BYPASS

- *Each year two people of every 1,000 in the U.S. have surgery on their coronary arteries. The majority of these have open heart operations for bypass grafts. In Canada (and other countries), fewer bypass surgeries are performed.*
- *If you have had a coronary artery bypass graft (using a vein taken from your leg to bypass an obstructed coronary artery), you run*

one chance out of two that the vein will become partly or completely plugged by atherosclerosis after 12 years. Preventive measures will reduce this risk.

■ SUMMARY

If you have any of the above listed controllable risk factors, your sense of freedom may be curtailed and your enjoyment of life may be affected. But there is much you can do to lessen these risks. Becoming informed about your heart attack risks, and learning how to reduce them, can give you greater self-confidence and a feeling of peace and accomplishment.

This book will show you how to minimize your risks, and so lead a longer, healthier, and more enjoyable life.

How Heart Problems May Affect You

2

If you have heart trouble, the physical effects may be completely without symptoms, or you may have symptoms. Other repercussions are psychological, social, and work-related.

SILENT HEART TROUBLE

Silent Heart Attacks

When you have a check-up that includes an electrocardiogram (EKG or ECG), you may be surprised to learn that the pattern shows definite evidence of a previous heart attack, about which you knew nothing. If you had no symptoms at all, you have had a silent heart attack. If you experienced unexplained "indigestion" with pain or discomfort in the upper abdomen, you have not had a silent heart attack but an "atypical" heart attack. About one in four heart attack victims has had an atypical heart attack.

It is possible to have a heart attack without any noticeable symptoms.

Probably fewer than one in ten heart attacks is truly silent. If you have diabetes, you will be more prone to a silent heart attack. They may also occur when a person is undergoing surgery or suffering from an injury.

Silent Exertional Ischemia

If you have coronary artery plaque (patches in the coronary arteries made of cholesterol deposits, and fibrous and muscle tissues) that partially blocks the blood flow to part of your heart muscle, the blood flow through the diseased artery may be quite adequate for resting conditions, but not for the increased demands of exercise. Exercise tests while patients are connected to an electrocardiogram often reveal that the blood flow through a part of the heart is inadequate for a certain amount of exertion. When this electrocardiographic change is seen without other symptoms it is called silent exertional ischemia.

If tests show that you have silent exertional ischemia, this is a warning that you are at risk for a heart attack. You and your doctor will need to develop a preventive strategy immediately.

HEART TROUBLE WITH PHYSICAL SYMPTOMS

Angina (Angina Pectoris)

Angina refers to the pain or discomfort, usually in the front of the chest, that accompanies insufficient blood flow through one or more coronary arteries. Often the pain will radiate to the left or right arm, or into the throat or jaw.

It usually subsides after a few minutes. If angina persists for more than 20 minutes, a heart attack is the likely cause, and you must call for emergency help. The main symptom of a heart attack (coronary thrombosis, or myocardial infarct) is angina. It sometimes persists for hours, but usually more than 20 minutes.

Atypical Angina

If the pain is not typical—that is, not in the chest or arms—it may still be heart pain. It may be felt in the stomach region, or the back of the chest or neck. The pain may even be felt as a toothache or an earache.

Angina may be mistaken for a stomachache or even a toothache.

If you have angina, whether typical or atypical, you will usually feel it while exerting yourself, and can relieve it within a minute or so by resting. If it persists for 20 minutes or more, you may be having a heart attack. Do not delay. Call for emergency help.

Shortness of Breath

Angina may be accompanied by shortness of breath or a feeling of suffocation. But sometimes shortness of breath may be the only symptom indicating that not enough blood is reaching your heart. This is more likely to occur in people over age 70.

Chronic, Stable Angina

If you can predict when your anginal distress will bother you, you have chronic, stable angina. For example, perhaps you can walk on level ground in comfort, but walking uphill causes chest pain, which is relieved when you stop. Chronic, stable angina may very slowly worsen. Last year it may have occurred only when you ran; now it may occur when you walk quickly. You may feel the discomfort at rest when you are emotionally upset. To be considered chronic and stable, however, the pain should be predictable in specific situations.

Unstable Angina

"Unstable angina" is unpredictable, requiring immediate medical attention.

If you cannot foresee under which circumstances you will have anginal discomfort, you have unstable angina. The pain may awaken you from sleep, or it could occur while you are relaxing. It may last 5 or 10 minutes; if it fails to subside spontaneously, you may be having a heart attack.

Unstable angina is a dangerous condition. If you suffer from unstable angina, you need urgent medical attention to prevent a heart attack.

Disorders of Heart Rhythm

If you feel your heart flipping or pounding (see p. 109), you are not alone. Many people are troubled with this feeling, but the majority are reassured after a check-up. In a few cases, however, these symptoms reflect the presence of ischemia (insufficient oxygen in heart tissues) due to coronary artery disease. For example, if you have had a recent heart attack and have a certain kind of heart irregularity known as premature ventricular contractions, you probably will need special attention to prevent further complications.

Congestive Heart Failure

If your heart is damaged from one or more previous heart attacks, longstanding high blood pressure, or other causes, you are at risk for congestive heart failure (insufficient circulation of blood throughout the body due to weakness of the heart muscle). When this condition is mild, it causes only shortness of breath upon extra exertion. If the condition worsens, the shortness of breath becomes more troublesome. In addition to breathing problems, the heart enlarges, ankles and legs swell, and internal organs, such as the liver, become congested. If the condition becomes more severe, you can expect to be more tired and have a poor appetite.

If you have congestive heart failure, you are at greater risk for other circulatory complications, such as heart attack or stroke. You will need careful prevention and treatment plans.

PSYCHOLOGICAL EFFECTS OF HEART TROUBLE

Heart trouble has very different psychological effects on different people, some of which are discussed on the following pages.

Fearfulness

You may feel fearful, insecure, and afraid of situations in which you need to exert yourself, or that cause you to get excited. As a result, you may limit your life experiences, avoiding physical exertion, emotional stress, and sexual activity.

The state of your heart is important for you not only physically, but emotionally and spiritually as well.

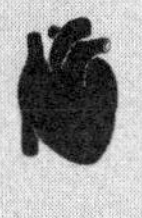

Insomnia may be a problem if you fear dying in your sleep.

You may become overdependent on medication. Your anxiety may make you reluctant to cut down or cancel medication even if your doctor suggests it. If changes are made in your medications you may find symptoms that convince you to resume the more familiar medications.

By realizing that these attitudes are common and that they are a natural result of fear, you can accept and overcome them. When you go for a check-up, discuss your fears with your doctor. You may discover that your heart function is better than you imagined.

Often a positive result of heart disease is a newfound enjoyment of everyday life.

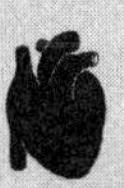

Heedlessness

You may become foolishly brave. Some people with heart conditions develop a kind of rash courage, challenging themselves excessively or taking unnecessary chances. If this is one of your traits, it is important for you to recognize that you are overcompensating from anxiety. True courage is reasonable; rash courage is potentially self-destructive.

Anger

You may become angry, knowing that you are vulnerable to the unexpected. You may feel indignant at being the victim. You then become irritable and can develop a chip on your shoulder. This attitude can make you feel jealous of those who are well.

Again, if you recognize that these feelings are normal, you can overcome them. Talking to your doctor or to someone who is close to you may also help.

Guilt

You may feel guilty that you have developed heart trouble. If you have not exercised regularly, or believe that you have not paid proper attention to your diet, or have smoked cigarettes, you could feel remorseful. This attitude is reinforced by society's focus on our personal responsibility for preventing heart trouble. But do not dwell on the past. Instead, make positive changes in your lifestyle now.

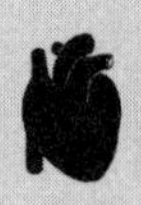

Focusing on the positive changes you can make is vital to your health and survival.

Hopelessness

You may feel pessimistic and hopeless, but this attitude is unproductive, since there is usually much to be hopeful about your condition. Try to focus on the positive, on what you *can* do rather than on what you cannot do.

Serenity

One of the unexpected benefits of having heart trouble is that you may become more mellow and philosophical as a result of it. Becoming aware of your fragility can cause your spirit to blossom. You can become softer and more compassionate. You may take the time to enjoy life, your family, and your friends. You may read more, do volunteer work, or become more spiritually aware. Your life can become richer and more meaningful.

Psychological Defenses

The fear of heart trouble may cause you to erect one or more psychological defenses. These may include denial, repression, projection, regression, or procrastination. If you have developed exaggerated defenses, you may need professional counselling to help you cope.

Psychological counselling is helpful for coping with a wide range of emotional reactions.

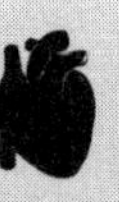

Are You A "Denyer"?

If you are a "denyer," you protect yourself from worry by just not admitting there is a problem. You act as if there were no problem. Obviously, this trait can be dangerous.

Are You a Represser?

If you are a represser, you bury your worries and fears; they are swallowed but not digested. Thus, you cannot deal with them effectively. This will cause an ongoing feeling of unease and discontent.

Are You a Projector?

If you lash out, blaming everyone else for your situation, you are a projector. It is too painful to admit that there is a fault within you, so you blame others, including your doctors. This will make it difficult for you to follow a good preventive program.

Are You a Regresser?

If your worry and anxiety cause you to become childlike and dependent, you are a regresser. In this case, you may feel that you need an authority figure, perhaps someone in your family or perhaps the doctor, to make decisions for you. You may seek many different sources for advice, ending up with a confusing array of treatments.

Are You a Procrastinator?

Perhaps you keep yourself so busy that you just don't have enough time to look after your own health. You know you should, but you are too preoccupied, and have put your good intentions on a shelf. You must prioritize your duties.

What could be more important than the care of your health?

Are You Well-Balanced?
If you are well-balanced, you can handle your anxieties in a mature and rational manner. You can put your priorities in order and take appropriate action.

Note: The theme of this book is change for the better. If your psychological defenses are inappropriate for your health and happiness (and the happiness of people close to you), remember that you *can* change. Seek a professional counsellor to help you develop more positive stress responses. (See SUGGESTED READING, especially *Heart to Heart.*)

HOW HEART PROBLEMS MAY AFFECT YOU SOCIALLY

If you develop a heart condition, your social life may show no change, or it may change radically. This will depend upon how the illness affects you both physically and emotionally. Your sexual function may or may not be affected. Problems with impotence and frigidity often occur with angina or after surviving a heart attack. (See p. 63–64.)

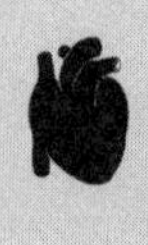

Simplifying a busy social schedule can have both physical and emotional benefits.

In your home and workplace, it is important for you and those around you to understand your strengths and limitations, so that no one will worry unnecessarily.

A serious heart condition may also have a serious effect on your financial state. If so, your social life will be affected. You and your family can benefit, however, by adopting a simpler lifestyle, and slowing the giddy pace that is so common today.

HOW HEART PROBLEMS MAY AFFECT YOUR WORK

If you have survived a heart attack, or if you have angina, your work life may be affected in some way. Even if your heart condition does not impair your ability to exert yourself, anxiety and depression about your heart could needlessly cause you to discontinue your work. You may find your memory and concentration impaired from stress, making it difficult for you to make decisions. This is likely a result of accumulated stress, related to "post-traumatic stress disorder," commonly known as "burnout syndrome." If you are experiencing difficulty with your work, you will probably benefit from professional counselling.

Heart patients often experience stress at work due to anxiety about their health.

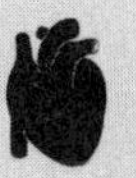

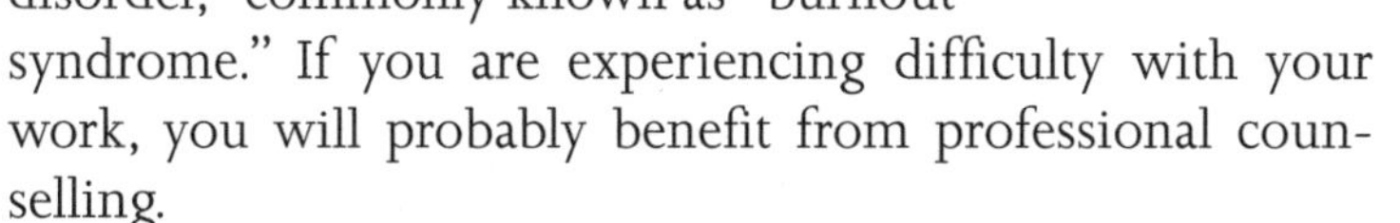

If you have had "successful" surgery to bypass obstructed arteries, it is possible you may choose not to return to the work force. When people do not, it is most commonly as a result of stress. (Statistics show that most people who return to work after bypass surgery were off work for a relatively brief time before surgery, or showed intentions of returning to work in the preoperative period.)

If you are given a choice between medical treatment or surgical bypass for your heart condition, you may believe that bypass surgery is more likely to restore you to a condition fit for work. However, in most cases, taking medications for angina has been shown to be just as effective as bypass surgery for keeping a person at work.

Being unable to work has both financial and psychological ramifications. You may have to cut down on expenses and simplify your lifestyle. You may also have to find new ways to spend your time and to give purpose to your life. These challenges offer you an opportunity for personal growth.

■ SUMMARY

If you have heart trouble, you may or may not have physical symptoms. You may also experience psychological, social, and work-related effects. Some of these effects may be beneficial, allowing you to enjoy a richer life, whereas others may seem negative. But it is quite possible to change these negative effects into positive effects.

A Medical Check-up for Your Risk Level

3

To find out if you are at risk for a heart attack, you must make an appointment for a check-up with a competent physician who has a good reputation for preventive cardiology. A check-up includes:

- *an interview with the doctor*
- *a physical examination*
- *several diagnostic tests*

DOCTOR/PATIENT INTERVIEW

Exploring Heart Symptoms

The doctor will want details of any discomforts in your chest, or in your arm or shoulder, that may reflect heart trouble.

- *Are these discomforts related to exercise? If so, the possibility that they are related to your heart increases.*
- *How long does the discomfort last?*
- *Is it associated with any other symptoms, such as shortness of breath, faintness, gas, or heartburn?*

Your answers to these questions can help your doctor determine whether your symptoms have a low, moderate, or high likelihood of being caused by your heart.

Your Family History

The doctor will need to know about your family history.

- *Is there a family history of premature heart attacks or other artery problems? Having a grandfather who died of a heart attack at age 80 is not worrisome, but if your father and uncle suffered heart attacks in their 40s or 50s, this would demand very careful attention, unless you have passed well beyond these age groups.*

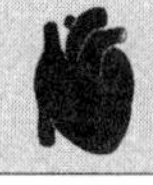

Some heart attack risk factors can be inherited.

- *Do any blood relatives have abnormal cholesterol, diabetes, or high blood pressure? These conditions in the immediate family increase your risk for heart attacks.*

Your Lifestyle

Your lifestyle will be reviewed by the doctor.

- *Do you smoke? If so, how much? If you have quit, was that yesterday or 10 years ago?*
- *What are your eating habits? A review of your typical breakfast, lunch, and dinner is helpful.*
- *Do you drink alcohol? If so, what type, how often, and how much?*
- *What has your weight pattern been in the past few years?*
- *What are your exercise habits?*
- *What are your working conditions and hours? Do you enjoy your job? How many hours a week do you work?*
- *What do you enjoy most in your life?*
- *When problems arise, what strengths have you found helpful?*

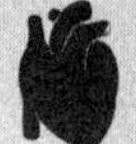

Lifestyle habits have a strong impact on heart disease.

■ THE DOCTOR'S PHYSICAL EXAM

Checking for Signs of Heart Trouble

During the physical exam your doctor will try to observe as many clues as possible that could betray a risk for heart trouble. These include:

- *xanthomata, small white or yellow cholesterol deposits on the skin near the eyes, or lumps on the tendons of the hands or feet*

- *gray circles in the colored portion of the eye (the iris) called "arcus senilis"*
- *creases of the lower part of the earlobes*
- *a "pot belly" (when the circumference of the waist exceeds that of the hips)*

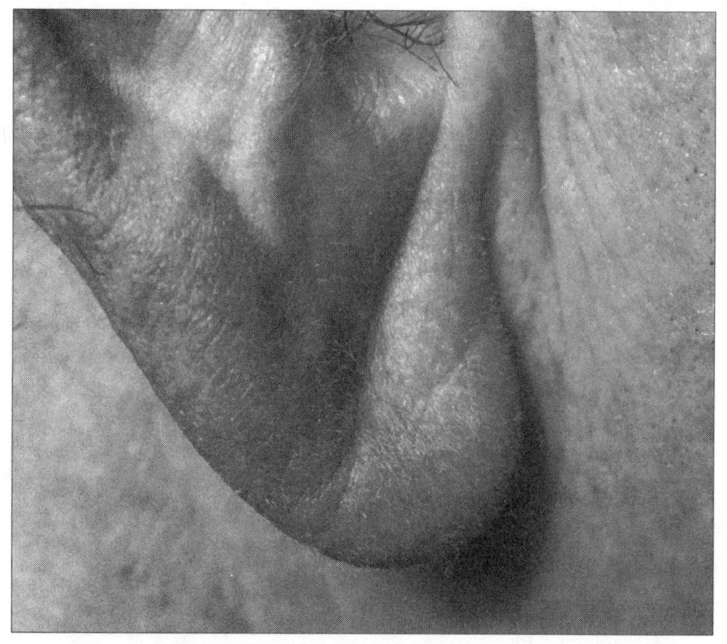

An earlobe crease like the one shown here may indicate heart attack risk.

Your Blood Pressure Reading

Your blood pressure will be carefully checked and rechecked. The reading shows the blood pressure in the two phases of the heartbeat, contraction and relaxation.

A diagnosis of high blood pressure is made only after several readings.

A typical normal blood pressure reading is 120 over 80 (usually written as 120/80). This means that the pressure in the artery of the arm (where the blood pressure cuff is applied) is enough to suspend mercury in a glass column at the 120-millimeter point. This is called the systolic pressure. The diastolic pressure (during the relaxation phase of the heartbeat) is enough to suspend the mercury column at 80 millimeters.

If your blood pressure is greater than 140/90 on repeated checks, you have high blood pressure. The diagnosis of high blood pressure will not be made on a single reading. Even on the same visit to the doctor the readings may vary 10 to 30 or more points.

Checking for Artery Disease (Atherosclerosis)

Do you have any direct signs of artery disease? To find out, your doctor can:

- *view the small arteries of your eye with a special instrument called an ophthalmoscope*
- *listen for a "bruit" over the carotid arteries of your neck and the iliac arteries in your groin. A bruit is a rough, pulsating sound heard when the stream of blood passes over a surface roughened from atherosclerosis. Normally the flow is quite silent, like a river flowing over a deep, smooth area. In contrast, where the riverbed is narrow and rough, the flow is quite audible.*
- *carefully feel the small arteries of your feet, where a faint or absent pulse may betray the presence of atherosclerosis*
- *examine your abdomen for signs of an aneurysm of the major artery, the aorta. An aneurysm is a bulging of an arterial wall weakened by atherosclerosis.*

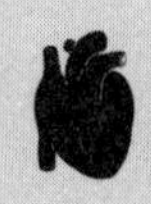

A doctor can detect signs of artery disease by listening to your blood flow.

Your doctor will also observe such things as how you respond to emotional stress, and whether or not you have signs of diabetes, thyroid disorder, lung conditions, or any other diseases that could have a bearing on your heart.

THE DIAGNOSTIC TESTS

Note: It is unlikely that any one person would be given all the tests described below. Your condition and ongoing research will determine your doctor's choice of tests.

Your Electrocardiogram

A regular part of your heart attack prevention check-up is the electrocardiogram (EKG or ECG). In this examination, metal electrodes are attached to your arms, legs, and chest while you rest quietly.

Your EKG pattern shows the currents of electric energy during the various phases of the heartbeat. Like your signature, your EKG pattern is distinctive. The wave form tends to be similar over the years unless it is changed by conditions that affect the heart. Your electrocardiogram pattern will fall into either a normal or an abnormal range, and can show the following:

> *EKG patterns are distinct for each person.*

- *presence or absence of any irregularity of the heart rhythm*
- *signs of previous or present interferences with blood flow*
- *signs of a previous heart attack*
- *signs that one or more of your heart chambers is enlarged*
- *thickening (hypertrophy) of the left ventricle muscles caused by high blood pressure. If your EKG shows hypertrophy, your risk for heart attacks is greater than if there were no such thickening.*

If you are a man with a resting EKG pattern known as "non-specific ST depression," you are at extra risk for a heart attack. The same pattern in women is not a risk factor.

Note: A normal EKG in no way means that your risk of a heart attack is low. Many heart attack victims have a normal EKG pattern immediately before a heart attack. Your EKG pattern is compared with later ones that may show abnormal features.

> *A normal EKG does not necessarily mean that your heart attack risk is low.*

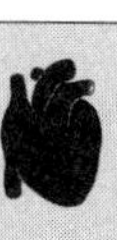

Your Chest X-Ray

An enlarged heart is a risk factor for heart attacks. A chest x-ray roughly shows the heart's dimensions, and is commonly used for this purpose.

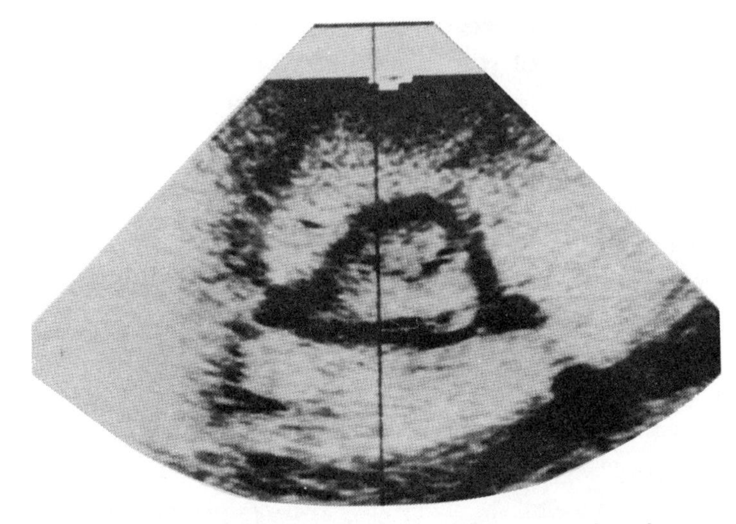

Ultrasound waves show your heart's size and shape in an echocardiogram.

Your Echocardiogram

Even more accurate for showing the size and shape of your heart's structures is the echocardiogram.

You lie on a table while a technician directs a flashlight-sized probe over your chest to send ultrasound waves through your heart. The pattern of these waves is interpreted by experts, who report their findings to your doctor. Some doctors conduct this test in their offices.

Your Blood Tests

Routine blood tests should include:

- *a hemoglobin test to rule out anemia, which may affect the heart by failing to deliver enough oxygen to the heart muscle*
- *blood sugar levels to determine whether you have diabetes*
- *blood lipid levels (your cholesterol and triglyceride counts)*

Measuring Cholesterol

In the U.S., cholesterol is measured in milligrams per deciliter (mg/dL). In Canada, cholesterol is measured in millimoles per liter (mmol/L).

If your cholesterol report is in millimoles per liter and

you want to translate it into milligrams per deciliter, you multiply the number of millimoles by 38.7. For example, 5.17 mmol/L × 38.7=200 mg/dL. If your report is in milligrams per deciliter and you want to translate it into millimoles per liter, divide the number of milligrams by 38.7.

Your blood should be tested for hemoglobin, blood sugar, and blood lipid levels.

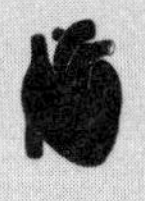

Your Cholesterol Report

Often a cholesterol report gives only the total cholesterol. A more complete report is often advisable, and includes the following:

- *total cholesterol*
- *high density lipoprotein (HDL) cholesterol*
- *low density lipoprotein (LDL) cholesterol*
- *triglycerides*
- *ratio of total cholesterol to HDL cholesterol*

Your Total Cholesterol Level	
Low risk	under 200 mg/dL (5.17 mmolL)
Intermediate risk	200–240 mg/dL (5.17–6.2 mmol/L)
High risk	greater than 240 mg/dL (6.2 mmol/L)

Your HDL ("good") cholesterol: The levels of HDL cholesterol in your blood should exceed 45 mg/dL (1.16 mmol/L).

Your LDL ("bad") cholesterol: The levels of LDL cholesterol in your blood should not exceed 130 mg/dL (3.36 mmol/L).

Your ratio of total to HDL cholesterol: The ratio of total cholesterol to HDL cholesterol has been found to be a better risk indicator than the total cholesterol level or the HDL cholesterol level alone. It is calculated by dividing the total cholesterol by the HDL cholesterol. Suppose your total cholesterol is 300 mg/dL and your HDL cholesterol is 75 mg/dL. Your ratio would be: 300 ÷ 75 = 4. (See also GLOSSARY.)

If your total cholesterol level is 300 mg/dL and your HDL cholesterol is only 37.5 mg/dL, the ratio would be expressed as: 300 ÷ 37.5 = 8.

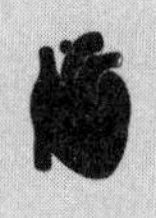

The ratio of total cholesterol to HDL cholesterol is an important risk indicator.

These ratios are, of course, the same when millimoles per liter (mmol/L) are used. When the ratio is above 4.5 for both women and men, the risk of a heart attack is greater than average.

Your triglyceride count: The normal range for triglycerides is 52–204 mg/dL (0.59–2.3 mmol/L). To change between the metric system and millimoles for triglycerides, you multiply (or divide) by 88.5.

The triglyceride count is often high when the HDL cholesterol is low and vice versa. If your triglyceride level is high and your HDL cholesterol level is low, your risk for a heart attack is especially high, even if your total or LDL cholesterol is low.

Here is a typical cholesterol report:

In millimoles per liter the same report would be:

Doe, John: Age 62 / Sex M / Date 19 Feb. 1995		
Lipid	Results	Normal Range
Cholesterol	205 mg/dL	160–240 mg/dL
Triglyceride	232 mg/dL	52–205 mg/dL
HDL Cholesterol	47 mg/dL	45–85 mg/dL
LDL Cholesterol	111 mg/dL	70–130 mg/dL
Ratio Total Cholesterol/HDL Cholesterol: 4.4		

Doe, John: Age 62 / Sex M / Date 19 Feb. 1995		
Lipid	Results	Normal Range
Cholesterol	5.29 mmol/L	4.13–6.20 mmol/L
Triglyceride	2.62 mmol/L	0.59–2.30 mmol/L
HDL Cholesterol	1.21 mmol/L	1.16–2.19 mmol/L
LDL Cholesterol	2.87 mmol/L	1.81–3.36 mmol/L
Ratio Total Cholesterol/HDL Cholesterol: 4.4		

Your Urinalysis Test

A specimen of your urine will probably be checked as part of the examination, to test for the possibility of diabetes, a risk factor for heart attacks. It will also be checked for albumin, another risk factor.

Your Exercise "Stress" Test

The "stress" in the test refers to the physical stress of exercise. It is not a dangerous test. This test helps to show whether you are at extra risk for heart attacks. You exercise on a stationary bicycle or a treadmill while your heart is being monitored by an electrocardiogram, and you exercise until:

> *An exercise stress test monitors your heart rate, EKG pattern, and blood pressure.*

- *your heart rate is close to its maximal rate, as estimated for your age, or*
- *you become short of breath, your legs get tired, you get dizzy, or*
- *your EKG pattern on the monitor shows signals that the exercise should be stopped, or*
- *your blood pressure reading, which is checked regularly, is either too high or too low.*

There are three important things that your doctor will be observing:

1. How long were you able to continue exercising? If you needed to stop this exercise within the first 3 minutes, you could be at extra risk for a heart attack.
2. Were you able to exercise enough to cause your heart rate to approach the near-maximal figure?
3. Were there any shifts in the ST segment of your electrocardiogram as a result of exercise, and compared with the pattern before exercise? (See diagram, p. 24.) If so, was this brief, such as at peak exercise only, or did it persist for more than one minute after rest? As well, a shift greater than 2 millimeters would be serious.

While this test is very useful, it is not perfect, and must be

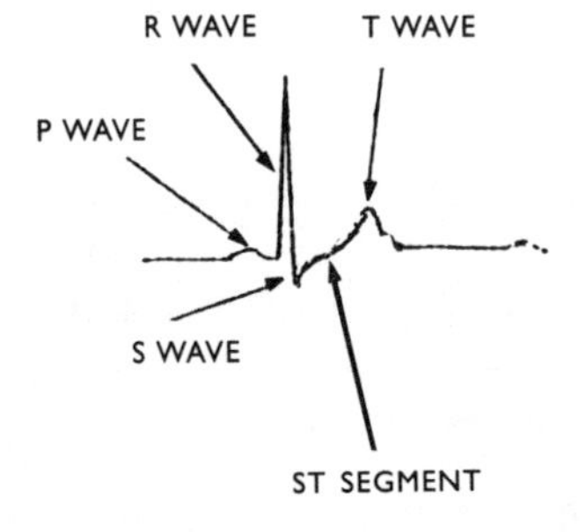

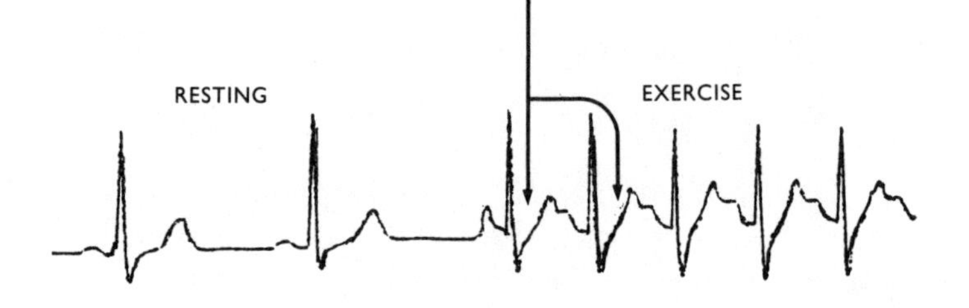

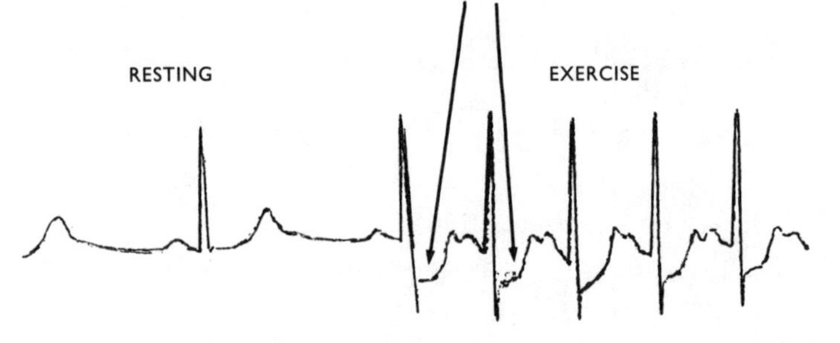

Waves of electrocardiogram, including ST segment

interpreted wisely, along with your other risk factors for a heart attack.

If you are under the age when heart attacks are common, and have no other risk factors for heart attacks, the exercise test is unlikely to provide useful information for you except reassurance that everything is normal. But if you are so worried about your heart that you fear exercise, you could benefit from receiving normal test results.

Unfortunately, a false positive reading may occur and is more likely when there are few risk factors. In this case ST segment shifts occur that mimic those which occur when coronary artery plaques reduce the blood supply for the exercising heart. To prove it is a false positive, you can repeat the exercise test, but with additional equipment and techniques. Two different procedures are available for this purpose: a mibi scan or an exercise echocardiogram.

The Mibi or Thallium Scan

Mibi (sestamibi) and thallium are substances that are rendered radioactive and injected in your vein while you are exercising. They are absorbed immediately by your heart muscle, where their radioactivity allows them to be detected by special equipment. (The amount of radioactivity that your body is exposed to during this test is no more than that of a common x-ray.)

A mibi or thallium scan can reveal coronary artery plaques.

If you cannot exercise, your doctor can obtain similar results by injecting dipyridamole along with the mibi or thallium. Dipyridamole dilates normal coronary arteries, reducing the flow down obstructed coronary arteries.

A sophisticated, computerized geiger counter shows the distribution of the mibi or thallium in the heart immediately after exercise, or after dipyridamole. This is compared with the distribution 3 or 4 hours later. If you have coronary artery plaques that interfere with blood flow during strenuous exercise, there will be less of the radioactive material in the muscles supplied by obstructed arteries.

The Exercise Echocardiogram

The exercise echocardiogram uses ultrasound waves to show the dimensions of the chambers of the heart as they contract and relax. If a portion of the heart fails to receive its needed supply of blood during exercise, this will show up on graphs taken immediately after exercise. After a few minutes, as the heart recovers from exercise, the graphs resume their pre-exercise shapes.

Dobutamine Stress Echocardiogram

If you are not able to exercise, an echocardiogram conducted before and after an injection of dobutamine has been found to be quite a reliable test to show signs of impaired coronary artery blood flow.

Dobutamine is a drug that mimics the effects of exercise: temporarily increasing the work of the heart by causing it to beat faster and against increased resistance. It must be given cautiously while you are connected to an electrocardiogram and your blood pressure is being monitored.

The Radionuclide Angiogram

This is a non-invasive test to analyze certain aspects of your heart's anatomy and function. You are connected to an electrocardiogram, which is linked to a gamma camera and computer. Radioactive technitium is injected intravenously, and attaches itself to your red blood cells. The camera will detect the radioactivity, to show the heart wall, or "wall motion abnormalities."

Ultrafast Computerized Tomography

A relatively new test can be used to help you find out if there are calcium deposits in your coronary arteries (a sure sign of atherosclerosis) by scanning the arteries in thin sections. It uses very little radiation, and is over in about 10 minutes. You do not need to exercise or receive any injections. However, this test does not reveal the degree of coronary artery obstruction. Sometimes highly calcified arteries may not obstruct blood flow.

The Coronary Angiogram

This test shows the internal diameters of the coronary arteries and the degree of narrowing of various points. A narrow tube is inserted into the femoral artery in the groin and passed up to the mouths of the coronary arteries. Dye is then delivered through the tube to these arteries at the same time as x-rays are taken.

Since this test is expensive and "invasive" (it involves a tube entering your arteries), if your doctor thinks you have coronary atherosclerosis, he or she will probably not recommend a coronary angiogram without first obtaining results from one or more of the tests described above.

A coronary angiogram is a final step in testing for artery disease.

AFTER YOUR CHECK-UP

Your check-up can tell where you stand compared with the average for heart attack risk for your age group and gender. With this information, you will know whether your heart attack prevention strategies need to be aggressive, or otherwise. If you are in a high risk group, you may be surprised to discover as you read on the dramatic benefit you can derive by aggressive management of your risk factors.

SUMMARY

If you think you may be at risk for a heart attack, you should have a check-up by a physician who is knowledgeable about preventive cardiology. This check-up should include an interview with the doctor, a physical exam, and diagnostic tests.

During the interview, the doctor should ask you about:

- *your symptoms of heart trouble*
- *your family history*
- *your lifestyle*

During the physical exam, the doctor should check for:

- *your blood pressure reading*
- *signs of heart trouble*
- *signs of artery disease (atherosclerosis)*

The diagnostic tests may include:

- *an electrocardiogram (EKG or ECG)*
- *a chest x-ray*
- *an echocardiogram*
- *blood tests, including a cholesterol report*
- *urinalysis*
- *an exercise stress test*
- *the mibi or thallium scan*
- *the exercise echocardiogram*
- *the dobutamine stress echocardiogram*
- *the radionuclide angiogram*
- *ultrafast computerized tomography*
- *the coronary angiogram*

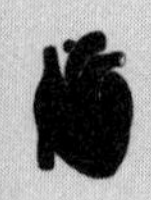

Ask your doctor if you do not fully understand your test results or their implications.

After your check-up, you should discuss the results and strategies for improvement with your doctor.

Assessing Your Own Risk Factors

4

THE MAJOR STATISTICAL RISK FACTORS

Your Blood Lipids

Levels of blood lipids (cholesterol and triglycerides) are the factors most commonly in need of improvement for heart attack prevention. They are also largely controllable through lifestyle management.

Statistical Facts About Cholesterol and Heart Attack Risks

- *If you are a man, your risk of heart attacks increases directly with your total cholesterol levels. If your cholesterol is less than 200 mg/dL (5.17 mmol/L) you are at low risk. If your cholesterol is 240 mg/dL (6.2 mmol/L) or more, you are at increased risk.*

A man with total cholesterol of over 240 mg/dL (6.2 mmol/L) is at higher risk of a heart attack.

- *If you are a woman, your heart attack rate is not increased unless your total cholesterol is very high, over 265 mg/dL (6.85 mmol/L).*
- *If you are taking birth control pills, you may expect to have a higher total cholesterol level (and higher blood triglycerides) than normal.*
- *Whether you are a man or a woman, your ratio of total cholesterol to HDL cholesterol is a more important risk factor than the*

cholesterol level itself. (See p. 21.)

- *If you are a woman or a man whose high total cholesterol is accompanied by low HDL cholesterol, you are at increased risk of a heart attack.*
- *Almost one in four men with high cholesterol also have high blood pressure, multiplying their risk of heart attacks.*
- *If you have high cholesterol, you are more likely to be overweight and sedentary, further increasing your heart attack risk.*

Your LDL ("Bad") Cholesterol

LDL cholesterol is the culprit in many heart attacks, because this fraction of the total cholesterol forms the deposits in the arteries affected by atherosclerosis. If you have a high total cholesterol level, the LDL cholesterol is likely to be responsible.

Your LDL cholesterol should not exceed 130 mg/dL (3.36 mmol/L). But if you have no evidence of coronary atherosclerosis, and no other risk factors, you do not need treatment for LDL cholesterol unless it is over 160 mg/dL (4.13 mmol/L).

If you are a middle-aged man, your LDL cholesterol will likely be higher than when you were younger. After age 35 or 40, most North American men have LDL cholesterol levels above normal. Women catch up to and pass men in this respect. Six in ten women aged 55 and over have abnormally high LDL cholesterol readings.

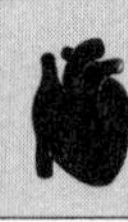

High levels of LDL cholesterol can result in artery plaque.

Your HDL ("Good") Cholesterol

HDL cholesterol is a reverse risk factor. It sweeps the arteries of cholesterol deposits, protecting them from atherosclerosis and preventing heart attacks. Women (especially before menopause) tend to have higher HDL cholesterol levels than men of the same age, averaging 55 mg/dL (1.42 mmol/L).

If you have a *low* HDL cholesterol, under 35 mg/dl (0.9 mmol/L), you are at risk for heart attacks even if your total cholesterol is low. If you have high levels of HDL cholesterol, you are at considerably less risk.

Low HDL cholesterol may be an inherited characteristic. As well, low HDL cholesterol levels are more common in cigarette smokers, or people who are overweight, with the fat around the waist rather than around the hips. If you have a physically active lifestyle, are lean and a nonsmoker, you are more likely to have higher HDL cholesterol.

HDL cholesterol helps to protect from artery disease.

Blood Triglyceride Levels

Triglyceride levels are often inversely related to HDL cholesterol because they inhibit its formation. If you have high blood triglycerides and a low level of HDL cholesterol, your heart attack risk is even greater than if you have one abnormal reading.

Most of the fats you eat are triglycerides. In addition, your liver can manufacture triglycerides. Excessive levels in the blood can result from both sources.

Your Family History

Genetically you may have extraordinary protection from heart attacks, or you may be dangerously vulnerable to them. Genetics can be responsible for:

- *high total and LDL cholesterols, without high triglyceride levels (familial hypercholesterolemia)*
- *high triglyceride levels with or without high cholesterol*
- *abnormally low HDL cholesterol, with or without raised LDL cholesterol or triglycerides*

All of these conditions make you vulnerable to heart attacks. If you have a family history of premature heart attacks (before age 55), you should have complete studies done of your blood lipids.

(The protein that carries HDL cholesterol is Apoliprotein A1 (Apo A1). Some families with a history of longevity carry this gene. Recently a mutation of it, Apo Milano, has been discovered, and genetically engineered versions have reversed plugged arteries in rabbits. This therapy may become useful for humans.)

If You Have High Blood Pressure

Facts About High Blood Pressure

- *Nearly two out of five adults have high blood pressure.*
- *High blood pressure is much more common after age 50.*
- *One in four people with high blood pressure is not aware of having it.*
- *If you have high blood pressure, your risk for heart attacks is greatly increased. For every 10 points that your blood pressure rises, your heart attack risk increases 30 percent.*
- *People with high blood pressure are also likely to have high cholesterol levels, to be overweight, and have a tendency to diabetes.*

How High Blood Pressure Can Lead to Heart Attacks

High blood pressure is caused by the difficulty of tiny arteries of the body to relax. It affects both the heart and the medium-sized arteries. Because the left ventricle of the heart must work harder to pump blood through the body, it gets thicker (hypertrophies). Its increased size and extra pumping effort causes it to need an increased blood supply from its coronary arteries.

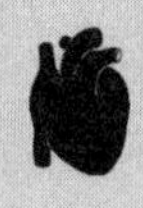

Pumping blood at a raised pressure is like riding a bicycle against the wind.

The inner surface of the arteries can then be damaged by increased blood pressure, and this damage triggers the atherosclerotic process. Since the medium-sized arteries are most affected, the heart's coronary arteries are vulnerable. The end result is that the diameter of the arteries is narrowed by atherosclerosis, yet these same arteries must provide more blood for the enlarged left ventricular muscle.

If You Smoke Cigarettes

Note: Pipe and cigar smokers do not have the increased heart attack risk of cigarette smokers. This is because if you smoke a pipe or cigar, you are unlikely to inhale the smoke, as many cigarette smokers do. If you do inhale cigar or pipe tobacco smoke, you are at increased risk just like cigarette smokers.

Smoking can inflate other heart attack risk factors.

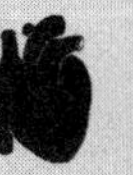

Facts About Cigarette Smoking

- *About one in three North American adults is a cigarette smoker. Fifty percent of smokers go through 20 or more cigarettes daily.*
- *Even moderate cigarette smoking (fewer than 20 per day) can inflate other mild or moderate risk factors to increase your risk of a heart attack greatly. For example, if your cholesterol is in the moderately high range and your blood pressure is only mildly above normal, smoking 10 to 15 cigarettes daily increases your heart attack risk 400 percent. Quitting cancels this risk, usually after a year or so.*
- *If you are a woman in your 40s who smokes and uses birth control pills, you are at greatly increased risk for a heart attack. (See Chapter 7.)*
- *If you are an older smoker and already have had some heart trouble, your risk for another heart attack (fatal or otherwise) is doubled.*

How Cigarette Smoking Can Lead to Heart Attacks

Cigarette smoking depletes your HDL (good) cholesterol levels. Twenty or more cigarettes daily reduces HDL cholesterol by up to 20 percent. Quitting permits your HDL level to rise. As well, cigarette smoke contains such toxic substances as carbon monoxide and nicotine, which may lead to artery damage and unwanted blood clotting.

If you are a cigarette smoker, be sure to have regular check-ups. Statistics show that smokers are more likely to have other heart attack risk factors: higher total cholesterol, higher blood pressure, a greater tendency toward diabetes. They also tend to be physically inactive—another risk factor.

Secondhand Smoke Hazards

- *Studies have shown that chemicals in secondhand, or "sidestream," tobacco smoke can injure the lining of the arteries, increasing the risk of death from heart disease 25 to 30 percent over that of people not regularly exposed to tobacco smoke.*

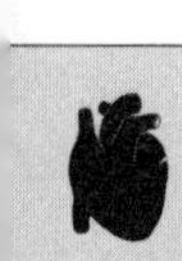

Secondhand smoke can severely damage your arteries.

- *The Environmental Protection Agency estimates that 53,000 nonsmokers die each year in the U.S. from the effects of secondhand cigarette smoke, up to 40,000 of them from heart disease.*
- *Secondhand smoke is the third leading preventable cause of death in the U.S., behind smoking and alcohol abuse.*

If You Use Illegal Drugs

Cocaine

Using cocaine for recreational purposes puts you at extra risk for heart attacks. Though this might be expected if you are already at risk for a heart attack, people with normal coronary arteries also die from cocaine-related cardiac arrest.

The drug quickens the heartbeat, and causes it to be erratic. At the same time, the heart must pump against a higher pressure due to the constricting effect of cocaine on the arteries. This also impedes circulation to the heart muscle. The result can be sudden cardiac death.

Marijuana

It is known that inhaling marijuana smoke increases the workload of your heart by raising your heartbeat and blood pressure. If you suffer from chronic, stable angina, smoking a marijuana cigarette will temporarily reduce your ability to exercise without pain.

If You Are Physically Inactive

Only about one in three adults in North America exercises regularly.

Being a member of the physically inactive majority places

you at just as much risk for a heart attack as any of the other major risk factors: high cholesterol, high blood pressure, or cigarette smoking. In fact, physical inactivity increases your risk for a heart attack two to four times.

■ OTHER RISK FACTORS

If You Are a Man

Until after age 50, being a man statistically increases your risk of having a heart attack. Differences between men and premenopausal women's HDL cholesterol levels are an important reason. Before menopause, women have higher HDL cholesterol than men.

Your Age

An important, unalterable risk factor for heart attack is age. For men, there is an almost 300 percent increase in the heart attack death rate in the U.S. population for those between the ages of 35 and 44 and those between the ages of 45 and 54. The rate increases relentlessly. For women, the disease kills just 12.5 people per 100,000 in the 35- to 44-year-old age group, but kills almost 1,000 per 100,000 of the 65- to 74-year-old age group.

The average age of a female heart attack victim is 9 years older than her male counterpart.

If You Are Overweight

Men who are 30 percent over their ideal weight have a 44 percent higher chance of dying from a heart attack; women have a 34 percent higher risk.

The Role of Triglycerides

If you are overweight, your blood triglyceride levels are probably above normal, especially if the weight is concentrated in the front, causing a paunch. This is more likely to be true if you are a woman past menopause or a man who is middle-aged or older.

Low HDL cholesterol and high blood pressure are often found together with a raised triglyceride count. In this situation, the raised triglycerides add still further heart attack risk to the effects of the other two.

If You Are Overweight at the Waist (Truncal Obesity)

If the girth of your waist exceeds that of your hips, you are more prone to heart disease than if the weight is carried on your hips. Statistics show that you are also then likely to have higher than normal blood pressure, higher cholesterol, triglyceride, and blood sugar (and insulin) levels, and lower than normal HDL cholesterol levels, all of which contribute to an increased risk of heart attack.

If You Are Very Stressed

Worry and a feeling of powerlessness can make you more vulnerable to heart attacks. Work overload and burnout are important factors in the cause of heart attacks, especially sudden cardiac death. Insomnia, which is often associated with stress, is a common complaint in patients with coronary atherosclerosis. If you have difficulty relaxing and impose rigorous schedules on yourself, you may be more vulnerable to heart attack.

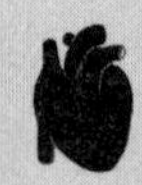

Stress itself is a heart attack risk factor.

There are different ways of handling stress. Studies show that if you feel overwhelmed and openly blow off steam, showing your anxiety or anger, you are less likely to suffer the inward effects of stress. In contrast, if you habitually appear cool and under control despite outward storms, you are more likely to suffer a heart attack. Although this likelihood may be related to raised blood pressure and cholesterol, both of which may rise with stress, these risk factors alone do not account for the bad effects of stress.

If You Have Diabetes (Diabetes Mellitus)

If you have diabetes, you need to take extra steps to protect yourself against the increased risk of heart attacks. (See SUGGESTED READING.) For example, if you are a woman with diabetes, your risk for a heart attack is increased threefold. But the risk catapults to sevenfold if you are a smoker with a high total cholesterol to HDL cholesterol ratio, and your blood pressure is above normal.

The heart attack risk is tripled for a woman with diabetes.

If You Have Type 1 or Type 2 Diabetes

Diabetes is a strong risk factor whether you have Type 1 (insulin-dependent diabetes mellitus—IDDM) or Type 2 (non-insulin-dependent diabetes mellitus—NIDDM). Type 2 is a risk factor even if it is only borderline.

Type 1 diabetes usually starts in childhood and tends to develop serious complications, such as diabetic coma, or excessively low blood sugar (hypoglycemia) as an overreaction to insulin injections.

Type 2 develops in adulthood, and may be controlled either by diet alone or diet in combination with antidiabetic pills. In Type 2 diabetes the pancreas produces too much insulin.

The Effects of Diabetes

Increased insulin in the blood increases the risk of heart attacks. Thus, the damage to the arteries in diabetes is due both to raised blood sugar and to raised levels of insulin.

With diabetes:

- *Your HDL cholesterol is lowered.*
- *Your LDL cholesterol is likely to be raised.*
- *Your ratio of total cholesterol to HDL cholesterol is raised.*
- *Your triglyceride level is raised.*
- *Your blood pressure is more likely to be raised.*

■ SUMMARY

You are at extra risk for future heart attacks if:

- *You are a man with high cholesterol levels.*
- *You are a man or a woman with a high ratio of total cholesterol to HDL cholesterol.*
- *You have low HDL cholesterol, even with a low total cholesterol.*
- *You have high blood triglycerides and you are a woman.*
- *You have high triglycerides and low HDL cholesterol, whether you are a woman or a man.*
- *You have high blood pressure.*
- *You smoke cigarettes.*
- *You are physically inactive.*
- *You are a man over 45.*
- *You are a woman over 55.*
- *You are overweight, especially if your extra weight is around your waist rather than around your hips.*
- *You are very stressed.*
- *You have diabetes.*

There is much that can be done to lower the risk of heart attacks, despite the presence of some unchangeable risk factors, such as aging. By improving those risk factors that you can work on, you can significantly improve your chances of being heart attack-free.

Reducing Your Risk Factors

5

Although you cannot control certain risk factors, such as your age, sex, and family history, you *can* strongly influence other risk factors. This chapter is about those risk factors, and how to reduce them.

■ SMOKING

Cigarette smoking is a potent risk factor at any age, but especially if you are under age 60. Decreasing the number of cigarettes you smoke to fewer than 10 daily reduces, but does not eliminate, your risk. (See also pp. 32–34.) You must *quit* smoking completely. There are some excellent books on this topic, such as *Detox*. (See SUGGESTED READING.)

As well, exposure to secondhand smoke increases your risk of heart disease significantly. If you live or work with smokers, you should avoid being exposed to their smoke. You have the right to demand a smoke-free work environment, and to ask smokers in your home to "light up" outside only.

■ LIPID LEVELS

Certain abnormalities of your blood lipids (cholesterol and triglycerides) will show that you are at extra risk for heart attacks. If you are a man, your total cholesterol is important. Whether you are a man or a woman, the ratio of your total cholesterol to HDL cholesterol is a valuable marker of your risk. The HDL cholesterol level, on its own, is also a reliable risk factor in either sex. If your ratio is above normal (4.5), you need to reduce the LDL content of your total cholesterol and maintain or increase the HDL content to improve the ratio.

If you have low HDL (good) cholesterol plus a raised triglyceride level, make every effort to correct this imbalance.

Most people can reach these goals by making several changes in lifestyle.

Increasing HDL Cholesterol

- *If you are a smoker, quit. Cigarettes reduce this beneficial cholesterol.* *(See p. 33.)*
- *If you are overweight, reduce. Losing pounds will increase your HDL cholesterol.*

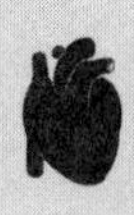

Weight loss and exercise will often increase your levels of HDL (good) cholesterol.

- *Exercise regularly. Most people can improve their HDL cholesterol with an exercise program. Even moderate exercise will increase the HDL cholesterol, but vigorous exercise will boost it more.*
- *If you have diabetes, good control of your blood sugar will help your HDL cholesterol.*
- *Ask your doctor about vitamin B_6 or vitamin B complex. If you are deficient in zinc, supplements may help increase your HDL cholesterol.*
- *Take vitamin C supplements, approximately 500 milligrams daily.*
- *Your doctor will advise you if medications such as niacin, or a fibric acid drug (either one of which may increase HDL cholesterol) should be used by you.*

Reducing LDL Cholesterol and Triglycerides

- *Watch what you eat and drink.*
- *Restrict your intake of dietary cholesterol. Egg yolks and organ meats are common sources of dietary cholesterol.*
- *Restrict your total fats and use unsaturated fats in moderation. Give priority to polyunsaturated omega 3 fats. (See p. 78.)*
- *Strictly limit your saturated (animal) fats. (See p. 77.)*
- *Be liberal with dietary fiber.*
- *Be moderate with your alcohol intake.*
- *Avoid regular use of decaffeinated coffee. In contrast to regular coffee, it can cause LDL cholesterol to rise.*
- *Eat garlic or onions for their beneficial effect on LDL cholesterol and the blood platelets.*
- *Take supplementary vitamin B complex and the antioxidant vitamins—C, E, and beta carotene—and selected trace minerals. (See p. 82.)*

  Vitamin B_6 and other B vitamins can raise HDL cholesterol in some cases. Antioxidant vitamins help keep LDL cholesterol from being dangerous. A deficiency in zinc can lower the HDL cholesterol. Supplementary chromium and magnesium may benefit your cholesterol levels. Magnesium also works with calcium and potassium to prevent artery spasm and control heart irregularities.
- *Enjoy foods rich in L-arginine, an amino acid found in nuts, seeds, and legumes. (See* APPENDIX, page 138.*) This precursor to nitric oxide is important for keeping your arteries healthy. Pumpkin seeds contain beneficial quantities of both L-arginine and alpha linoleic acid, the omega 3 fatty acid. Each seed contains only one calorie.*
- *Protect yourself from stress by learning effective techniques for stress control. Stress can worsen your cholesterol levels.*

■ HIGH BLOOD PRESSURE

High blood pressure is a common, serious malfunction that is responsible for many premature heart attacks and deaths. If you have only mild rises of blood pressure, you can usually bring about normal levels through changes in your lifestyle. Moderate or severe elevation of your blood pressure is best handled by making the same lifestyle changes, together with suitable medication prescribed by your doctor.

Grading High Blood Pressure

If you have high blood pressure, remember that your blood pressure level will vary somewhat from hour to hour, and day to day. Since blood pressure readings vary it is important to make decisions based on an *average* of several readings rather than on a single one. An average of your blood pressures will show whether you have mild, moderate, or severe high blood pressure. (See also p. 17.)

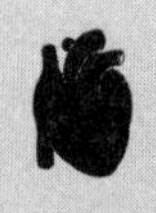

You can often regain normal blood pressure levels by making lifestyle changes alone.

	Mild	Moderate	Severe
Systolic blood pressure	141–160	161–199	200 or more
Diastolic blood pressure	91–104	105–114	115 or more

Use the following strategies to help you control your blood pressure.

- *Control your weight.*

  If you are overweight and have high blood pressure, make losing weight your top priority.

- *Eat less sugar.*

  Sugar has been shown to cause rises of blood pressure. If your blood pressure is high, cut down on sugar, honey, molasses, and the foods that contain them. (See SUGGESTED READING).

- *Eat less saturated (animal) fat.*

  Minimizing butter and other dairy fats, fatty meats, and coconut and palm oils can lower your high blood pressure. Vegetarian diets that include low-fat dairy products have been found to be beneficial for high blood pressure.

- *Use unsaturated fats (vegetable oils) in moderation.*

Moderate use of these oils may have a beneficial effect on your blood pressure readings. Canola oil, olive oil, safflower oil, sunflower oil, and corn oil are all good choices.

➠ *Eat more fish, or take fish oil supplements, providing at least 1,000 milligrams daily of eicosapentoic acid (EPA).*

Omega 3 fatty acids, which are found in the flesh of certain fish, can lower your blood pressure by as much as 10 points. (See p. 78, and *Seafoods and Fish Oils in Human Health and Disease* in SUGGESTED READING.)

Fish oils can help lower blood pressure levels.

➠ *Eat more fiber.*

Following a diet high in fiber, which is found in some fruits, vegetables, and grains, tends to lower blood pressure.

➠ *Limit your intake of wine, beer, or distilled liquor.*

One or two drinks a day may help lower your blood pressure, but increased amounts have the opposite effect. (See *Taking Control of Your Blood Pressure* in SUGGESTED READING.)

➠ *Eat less salt.*

We in the industrialized world eat about five times more salt than our bodies need, which is around 2.5 grams (.09 ounces) per day. Most of it is in processed foods. Even if you cut out salt in your cooking, and do not add salt to your food, you may still be taking in excessive salt hidden in prepared foods. (See *Food Values of Portions Commonly Used* in SUGGESTED READING.)

➠ *Get adequate amounts of trace minerals.*

Deficiencies of some trace minerals may be connected to high blood pressure. Certain trace minerals influence lipids and are discussed in the section on lipid levels, above. Although their benefits for high blood pressure are not yet conclusive, if your blood pressure is raised, try to get adequate amounts of calcium, potassium, selenium, magnesium, and zinc.

➠ *Guard against lead poisoning.*

If you have high blood pressure and have also been exposed to high concentrations of lead, get checked for the (rather remote) possibility that your raised blood pressure is due to mild lead poisoning. Lead is the most common toxic metal in the human body and usually comes from inhaling lead fumes or lead-containing dust. It may also be swallowed in food, often from unwashed hands, or in contaminated drinking water. Your blood lead level will show if you have lead poisoning. (See About Chelation Therapy, pp. 73–74.)

- *Exercise regularly.*

  Moderate exercise lowers blood pressure significantly. More vigorous exercise reduces it even more. (See *Take Heart!* in SUGGESTED READING.)

- *Manage your stress.*

  Improve your blood pressure with stress-reducing practices, which include regular exercise, relaxation, yoga, and meditation. (See *A Little Relaxation* in SUGGESTED READING.)

■ OBESITY

A support group can be very helpful when you are trying to lose weight.

Obesity—especially if the fat is around your waist rather than your hips—is bad for your heart. It is usually linked to lower HDL cholesterol, high triglycerides, and increased insulin levels.

Most overweight people are trying, or have tried, to lose weight. To succeed, you must:

- *Exercise regularly.*

  Daily exercise is an important way to prevent and combat obesity.

- *Drink lots of pure water or healthy, calorie-free drinks, such as unsweetened, mild herbal teas.*

  Drinking calorie-free fluids helps you feel full.

- *Cut down on fats.*

  Fats have twice the calories per gram as proteins or carbohydrates.

➠ *Eat less sugar.*

Sugar calories are often called "empty," since sugar lacks beneficial nutrients such as vitamins, minerals, and fiber.

➠ *Use alcohol wisely.*

If you drink alcohol, be moderate. Every ounce of alcohol has 198 calories (7 calories per gram), making it a significant contributor to obesity. Alcohol may also increase your appetite and lower your resolve to eat less.

Note: To calculate the calories in an amount of alcohol, you can use the following equation: 0.8 × proof × ounce. (Proof: 2 × the percentage of the alcohol content.)

For example, to calculate the calories in 8 ounces of wine containing 12 percent alcohol:

0.8 × proof × ounce. (Proof = 2 × the percentage of alcohol content).
12 × 2 = 24 proof.
0.8 × 24 × 8 = 153.6 calories.

(From "Alcohol and Calories," C.F. Gastineau. Mayo Clinic Proceedings, 1976 51 (2) 88.)

➠ *See also* SUGGESTED READING.

PHYSICAL EXERCISE

You can reduce your heart attack risk by exercising regularly. (See pp. 51–52, and 83–87.) At the same time you will find an improvement in your general well-being.

BLOOD CLOTTING

You can cut down your chances of having a heart attack by keeping your blood in a state where it is less likely to clot.

➠ *If you have two or more risk factors for heart attacks, speak to your doctor about taking low-dose coated or buffered aspirin. Even one-quarter of a 325 mg aspirin tablet is enough.*

Aspirin can reduce heart attack risk, and is safe for most people.

This simple treatment has been shown to have remarkable results in preventing heart attacks, by lubricating blood platelets.

But, if you are allergic to aspirin, or if this low dose causes indigestion, beware of this treatment. In a few cases it can cause stomach bleeding. If this is a problem, your doctor may prescribe an anti-clotting medication which does not irritate the stomach.

- *A diet including eicosapentoic acid (EPA) from fish oil, garlic, onions, and a moderate alcohol intake can also reduce your chance of having blood clots.*
- *Losing excess fat and getting regular exercise are also important in preventing blood clots.*

STRESS

Stress is known to raise cholesterol, triglyceride, and blood pressure levels. It can make someone with heart disease more vulnerable to sudden cardiac death. (See pp. 87–88 for some stress management techniques.)

DIABETES

If you have diabetes, reduce your risk factors for heart disease by controlling your diabetes, and following the strategies described throughout this chapter. (See also SUGGESTED READING.)

- *If you have Type I (insulin-dependent) diabetes, your doctor will help you control your blood sugar level with insulin therapy. Getting enough insulin can improve your HDL cholesterol and your ratio of total cholesterol to HDL cholesterol.*
- *If you have Type 2 (non-insulin-dependent) diabetes, you can help keep your blood insulin levels low by controlling your weight and exercising. Do not rely on your diabetic pills to do the job for you. Although they lower your blood sugar, they do not help your blood insulin.*

KEEPING INFORMED

Stay informed about your personal risk factors, and keep a personal chart for yourself, like the Progress Chart in Chapter 11. You should also find out about the latest research on heart attack prevention by doing the following:

- *Ask your doctor questions. You are entitled to all pertinent an-*

swers. But respect your doctor's schedule.

- *Study related information sources at the public library, or buy suitable books. (See* SUGGESTED READING.*)*
- *Subscribe to periodicals such as* The Townsend Letter for Doctors, *911 Tyler St., Port Townsend, WA 98368-6541;* Newsletter, *The National Heart and Diabetes Treatment Institute Inc., 18800 Florida St., Huntington Beach, CA 92648.*
- *Join or establish a group with others who have a common interest in heart attack prevention.*

SUMMARY

Staying up to date on treatments and research will help you control your own preventive program.

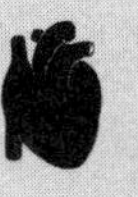

Follow these guidelines to control your heart attack risk factors:

- *If you are a cigarette smoker, quit.*
- *If you are exposed to secondhand smoke, do your utmost to avoid exposure.*
- *Know your blood pressure, and follow this chapter's guidelines to help keep it normal.*
- *Know your cholesterol ratio and triglyceride levels, and follow this chapter's guidelines to help keep them in the normal range.*
- *Control your weight.*
- *Eat fish two or three times a week. Or, consider taking fish oil supplements.*
- *Enjoy foods rich in L-arginine.*
- *Exercise regularly and sensibly.*
- *If you use alcohol, be moderate.*
- *Reduce your stress level.*
- *Take low-dose coated or buffered aspirin, if appropriate.*
- *Take daily supplements of vitamin C, vitamin E, beta carotene, and a vitamin B complex.*
- *Don't overlook the possibility of a lack of important trace minerals, such as zinc, chromium, selenium, magnesium, and others.*
- *If you have diabetes, emphasize all of the above, and take good care of your diabetes.*
- *Keep informed about the health of your own heart, and about the latest progress in heart attack prevention.*

6 If You Are Over Sixty

The numbers of older people continue to increase in North America. People over 65 now amount to 12 percent of the population, and in the coming decades this percentage will increase. If you are in this age group, you are three times more likely to die of heart disease than of cancer. Seventy-five percent of all deaths in people over 65 are due to heart attacks or heart failure. And disability as a result of heart attack or complications from a heart attack is very common among older people. These facts emphasize the need for prevention.

As you get older, the relative importance of the risk factors for heart disease changes. Some risk factors become less important, and some become more important.

■ YOUR FAMILY HISTORY

If one of your parents or an uncle died prematurely from a heart attack, your family history weighs heavily on you when you are young. But if you have survived to 65, your family history has no significance. However, your genes may positively affect your longevity if there is a family history of living to an old age.

■ IF YOU SMOKE

Statistics suggest that cigarette smoking becomes less of a risk factor for heart attacks after the age of 60. However, lung cancer or chronic obstructive lung disease (emphysema) can still ruin the health and life of a smoker whose habit has seemed safe for 60 years.

■ YOUR NUTRITION

Older people tend to have vitamin and mineral deficiencies. (See APPENDIX for further information.)

Vitamin B_{12} and Folic Acid

A new report from a long-term heart study revealed a surprisingly high incidence of latent Vitamin B_{12} deficiency in seniors, often despite using usual vitamin supplements. This, or folic acid (another member of the Bs) deficiency may be important. If you are over 60, and have signs of artery disease, speak to your doctor about taking 500 to 1,000 micrograms of B_{12} daily. This may be wise even if your serum B_{12} levels are in the normal range. Folic acid deficiency is less common.

Vitamin C

Vitamin C supplements can improve your HDL cholesterol levels and help you to ward off heart attacks. A new study supports the value of adding about 500 milligrams per day of vitamin C to your diet for heart attack prevention.

■ YOUR CHOLESTEROL LEVELS

Your cholesterol levels are still significant after age 60.

Cholesterol abnormalities continue to be important after age 60, though control of cholesterol levels takes second place to blood pressure control. HDL cholesterol is especially important for older people of both sexes.

Small HDL cholesterol level differences can have a significant impact on your chances for a heart attack. If you are 60 or over, increasing your HDL cholesterol by only 10 percent can mean the difference between suffering from heart disease and being free from heart trouble.

YOUR BLOOD PRESSURE

High blood pressure becomes more common as people get older. More than 40 percent of North Americans over 65 have high blood pressure. Men and women are equally affected. However, if you are black you may be especially vulnerable to high blood pressure; over 60 percent of black people over age 60 have high blood pressure.

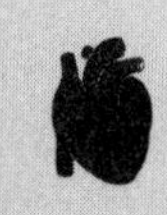

High blood pressure is the most common risk factor for older people.

Your Systolic Blood Pressure Reading

After age 65 the systolic blood pressure (the top of the two readings) becomes the important risk factor. Thus, a reading of 170 over 70 increases your risk of heart attacks, even though your diastolic blood pressure (the lower reading) is normal. This does not mean that you should ignore high diastolic levels, since the risk of heart attack for older people with raised diastolic blood pressure (e.g. 150 systolic, 120 diastolic) is reduced when high diastolic levels are treated.

Treating High Blood Pressure

If you are over 60, treating even mild high blood pressure can reduce your risk of heart attacks and other circulatory complications. Managing your blood pressure, for prevention, is a priority for your doctor.

A significant number of lives may be spared by treating high blood pressure in older people. However, some quite elderly patients who have had high blood pressure for many years cannot tolerate medicinal treatment. They may experience such symptoms as general fatigue and depression, memory loss, confusion, and unsteadiness. If you belong in this group, it is a good idea to ask your doctor to moderate the treatment or to consider abandoning it.

DO YOU EXERCISE?

Physical inactivity is often linked to aging and is encouraged by labor-saving devices and technology that favor sedentary lifestyles. Such habits as watching television or getting around the golf course in a motorized cart thwart physical fitness. In the many years that I have been conducting exercise "stress" tests, it is an infrequent but pleasurable experience to encounter an older person who is "fit."

Heart Health Benefits of Exercise

Regular exercise:

- *schools your heart to conserve energy, pumping more slowly and efficiently, with less demand on your heart arteries*
- *expands your coronary arteries and encourages a better blood flow in your heart muscle*
- *helps to prevent or control obesity*
- *helps to reduce raised blood pressure*
- *boosts your* joie de vivre *and helps combat depression*
- *reduces blood triglycerides, supports your HDL cholesterol, cuts the chances for harmful blood clots*
- *reduces your chances for sudden cardiac death and for heart attacks*

Staying physically active as you age may be your best insurance against heart disease.

It does not take much regular exercise to replace fat in the muscles with lean tissue. This in itself will improve your tolerance for exercise.

Finding a Suitable Form of Exercise

For people over 60, a walking program is safe, inexpensive, and easy to organize. And it is effective if you avoid walking at a slow stroll. You may prefer a stationary bicycle, but this type of equipment often falls into disuse. Swimming and dancing are excellent exercises, although they require considerable organization to become steady habits.

If you have arthritis in your lower extremities, swimming would be the preferred exercise.

Remember to check with your doctor before you embark on any type of exercise program.

SUMMARY

If you are over 60, some risk factors become more important and others become less important.

- *Maintaining normal blood pressure becomes the primary strategy in preventing heart disease.*
- *Second to that is improving your cholesterol levels, especially to keep the ratio of your total cholesterol to HDL cholesterol under 5, at least, and preferably under 4.*
- *Realize the value of suitable food supplements such as vitamin B_{12}, folic acid, and vitamin C.*
- *Family history also has less significance for your heart attack risk.*
- *Regular exercise remains important. The main purpose of avoiding a heart attack is to add quality time to your life. People who remain physically active are more likely to avoid depression, and to enjoy life with a sense of freedom and relative independence.*

If You Are a Woman

7

FACTS ABOUT WOMEN AND HEART DISEASE

- *If you are an American woman under the age of 45, you are ten times less likely to suffer a heart attack than your male counterpart.*
- *After menopause, when your risk of heart attack increases, you are half as likely as a man to have a heart attack.*
- *Nevertheless, heart disease is the major cause of death of older women, more prevalent than all cancers combined.*
- *For women, heart attacks tend to be more lethal; more women than men die with their first attack.*

YOUR RISK FACTORS AND WHAT YOU CAN DO

Your HDL Cholesterol

One apparent reason that women are protected from heart attacks is that they tend to have higher HDL cholesterol than men. HDL cholesterol, a powerful protector against heart attacks, is increased by the female sex hormone, estrogen. If your ovaries are functioning, you will probably have a higher HDL cholesterol level than the average male. Yours will likely be in the range of 55 mg/dL (1.42 mmol/L), while the average man's will be 45 mg/dL (1.16 mmol/L).

This difference in HDL levels accounts for the profound difference in the heart attack rate.

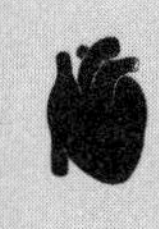

Naturally higher levels of HDL cholesterol give pre-menopausal women protection against heart attacks.

If you are a woman with abnormally low HDL cholesterol, you are 12 times more likely to suffer a heart attack than other women your age with normal HDL cholesterol.

➠ *Find out your HDL cholesterol level. If it is low, take the steps described on p. 40 to raise it.*

Your Total Cholesterol and LDL Cholesterol

A moderately high total cholesterol is less of a threat for women than for men. If your total cholesterol is 265 mg/dL (6.85 mmol/L) or less, chances are you do not need to worry. Similarly, a mildly elevated LDL cholesterol is less of a threat if you are a woman. As long as your HDL cholesterol is high, you do not need to worry about mild to moderate rises of your total and LDL cholesterol.

Your Ratio: a Valuable Predictor

Since HDL cholesterol is more important than the total cholesterol, but total cholesterol still has some significance, the ratio of the two has been found to be a useful predictor of future heart health. A total cholesterol to HDL cholesterol ratio of 4.5 indicates an average risk. A more favorable ratio is less than 4.

Your Triglyceride Levels

For men, an elevated triglyceride level is not a risk factor unless it is associated with low HDL cholesterol. For women, however, triglyceride levels above the normal range (177 mg/dL or 2.0 mmol/L) are an independent heart attack risk factor. This means that even if your ratio of total cholesterol to HDL cholesterol is normal, elevated triglyceride levels in the blood pose a heart attack risk.

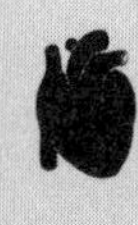

High triglyceride levels are more serious for women than for men.

A high triglyceride level is most worrisome when it is combined with other heart attack risk factors. If your triglycerides are elevated, you should try to keep your cholesterol ratio at 3.5 or less by minimizing your total cholesterol and raising your HDL cholesterol. You should also refrain from smoking cigarettes, and try to maintain a normal blood pressure.

You can lower triglyceride levels by reducing your calorie and fat intake, and by exercising.

What Will Cause Your Triglycerides to Rise

- *high calorie, high fat diet (except fish fat)*
- *alcohol consumption*
- *inactivity*
- *gaining weight*
- *having passed menopause*
- *taking the birth control pill*
- *diabetes*
- *kidney disease*
- *liver disease*

How to Lower Your Triglyceride Level

- *If you are overweight, lower your weight by reducing calories, especially saturated and vegetable fat calories, and by exercising. (See p. 41.)*
- *Avoid consuming alcohol.*
- *If you are on the birth control pill, discuss other options with your doctor.*
- *If you have diabetes, control your blood sugar by exercise and diet and, if necessary, such medication as insulin or diabetic pills.*
- *Add fish oil, which has potent triglyceride-lowering properties, to your diet either by eating a high fish diet or taking fish oil supplements. (See p.78.)*

If these procedures fail, and your risk warrants it, you may need medication such as niacin or a fibric acid agent. (See Chapter 9.)

Taking Birth Control Pills

Birth control pills (oral contraceptives) contain two hormones: progesterone and estrogen. The strength of either hormone varies according to the brand. If the pill has a high percentage of progesterone, it will tend to raise the LDL cholesterol, lower the HDL cholesterol, increase the HDL to total cholesterol ratio and raise blood pressure. In contrast, if the pill contains mostly estrogen, it has a more beneficial effect, including raising the HDL cholesterol.

If you take birth control pills *and* you smoke, you are at much higher risk for a heart attack. This risk is greatest if you are over 45. But even between the ages of 35 and 45, the risk of dying unexpectedly if you are on the pill and you smoke is well above normal for that age range.

If You Smoke

More women are smoking than ever before, and they are starting at an earlier age. Women need to be concerned about this, as they may be even more vulnerable to the effects of smoking than men.

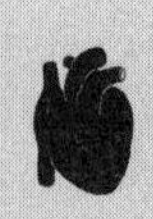

If you are over 45, smoke, and take birth control pills, you are at about the same risk of dying as a soldier in a battle zone.

The risk of heart attack is three times greater for the female smoker than for her nonsmoking counterpart. Even if you choose cigarettes with reduced nicotine, your risk does not improve.

If you quit smoking, within a couple of years your risk becomes about the same as that of women who have never smoked.

Dealing With Stress

If you are under excessive stress, you are at increased risk for heart attacks. Statistics show that if you are a married or single mother and are working at a job in which you play a subservient role, you could be at twice the risk for a heart attack as other women.

Many women carry responsibilities not only for their own children but also for their parents. This combination of responsibilities may interfere with healthful, leisure-time activities, and with opportunities for relaxation. The result is a feeling of being trapped, and of struggling against interminably oppressive circumstances. This pressure is an important contributor to heart attacks in women.

To combat the damaging effects of stress, it is important that you adopt effective stress management techniques. (See pp. 87–88.)

Stress is often a serious risk factor for women.

Estrogen Replacement Therapy

If you are at higher than average risk for heart attacks and are no longer menstruating—either because you have passed menopause or because you have had your ovaries removed—estrogen replacement medication can reduce your heart attack risk. Consult your doctor to make sure that there are no reasons not to take it, such as a history or a strong risk of breast cancer. Estrogen replacement therapy raises the HDL cholesterol, which tends to drop after menopause, and thus helps prevent heart attacks.

Estrogens are available and absorbed by skin patches as well as by pills (and also by injections). To prevent heart attacks, use pills instead of patches, since HDL cholesterol levels have not been shown to rise when patches are used.

Estrogen supplements may be helpful if you are postmenopausal and at risk for a heart attack.

Low-Dose Aspirin

If you are a woman at risk for heart attacks, check the use of low-dose aspirin for its important anticlotting effects. (See pp. 45–46 for details.)

If You Have Diabetes

The relative safety from heart attack that being a woman bestows is largely wiped out if you have diabetes. A diabetic woman is three times more likely to suffer a fatal heart attack than women of the same age who do not have diabetes.

This risk is even greater if you have other risk factors for heart attack. If diabetes is combined with high blood pressure, lipid abnormalities, or smoking, this greatly aggravates your risk. Unfortunately, if you have Type 2 (non-insulin-dependent) diabetes, you are more likely to have high

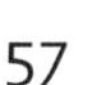

blood pressure and lipid abnormalities. Having these common extra risk factors will increase your heart attack risk to seven times the normal.

To minimize your heart attack risk if you have diabetes, include vigorous control of all risk factors, along with proper control of your diabetes. (See p. 46 for more information.) Don't forget the value of regular exercise if you have diabetes.

■ SUMMARY

If you are a woman at risk for heart attacks, follow these strategies:

- *Don't wait for heart trouble to strike. Know your risk factors and control them.*
- *Find out what your HDL cholesterol level is. Aim for 55 mg/dL (1.42 mmol/L). If your HDL cholesterol level is lower than this, the first step is to try to raise it through diet, exercise, and stress management techniques.*
- *Know your ratio of total cholesterol to HDL cholesterol. Aim for a ratio of less than 4.*
- *If your triglycerides are high, lower them. Meanwhile, maintain a cholesterol ratio of 3.5 or less.*
- *Maintain normal blood pressure.*
- *Lose weight if you are overweight.*
- *If you are on the birth control pill, consider other options.*
- *Don't smoke.*
- *If you are under stress, set aside time for exercise, meditation, or other stress management techniques.*
- *Consider taking estrogen replacement therapy if you are at risk for heart attacks and are no longer menstruating.*
- *If appropriate for you, take low-dose aspirin, to reduce your risk of heart attacks.*
- *If you have diabetes, control your blood sugar levels through diet, exercise and, if necessary, medication such as insulin or diabetic pills.*

If You Have Had a Heart Attack

8

If you have been discharged from hospital after suffering a heart attack, you are among the lucky minority. (Well over half of heart attack victims die within a month of the attack, most before they can reach a hospital.)

■ YOUR RISK GROUP

Your chances of developing serious complications over the next year depend on which of the following three risk groups you fall into.

- *Low Risk: One in three survivors of a heart attack is in the low risk group. If you fall into this group, you can expect to be relatively free from complications. You have a 98 percent chance of surviving the next 12 months.*
- *Intermediate Risk: About a quarter of recent heart attack survivors fall into this group. If in this group, you will need special treatment to help safeguard your chances of feeling well and surviving over the short term. Your chances of surviving the next year range between 97 percent and 75 percent.*
- *High Risk: These heart attack survivors, many of whom will be over age 70, have poor prospects of surviving the next few months. But they can beat the odds by rigorous control of their risk factors.*

Four factors determine which group you fit into:

- *the extent of damage to your heart muscle as a result of the heart attack*
- *the stability of your heartbeat. If your heartbeat tends to be irregular due to irritability of the damaged ventricle, there is increased risk of serious complications, at least within the first three months after a heart attack.*
- *the potential likelihood of further closures of either the same coronary artery that caused the first attack, or any of the remaining coronary arteries*
- *your attitude. Feeling depressed and morose, without hope, has a negative influence on survival rates. Feeling cheerful and optimistic has been found to have a positive effect on your chances for survival.*

If you are not in the low risk group, your doctors should assess whether you need to have coronary artery intervention, either by inserting a tube to open the obstruction (angioplasty) or bypassing the obstruction (coronary artery bypass graft). But in either case, you must prevent later problems by working to improve your risk factors.

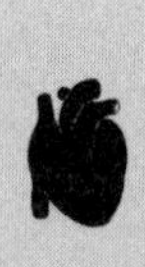

Even if you have had a heart attack, you can help prevent future trouble by making changes to your lifestyle.

No matter what risk group you fall into, remember, there is much that can be done with the help of modern medicine. You should also remember that a longer life is not your only goal; you want to enjoy good health and relative independence too.

STEPS FOR ACHIEVING YOUR GOALS

Taking Control of Your Life

Having a heart attack is a severe blow physically, psychologically, and socially. For many, this adversity offers an opportunity for renewal, a greater appreciation of life, and the realization that you need to take more control over the things that affect you. Many heart attack survivors enjoy further years of a good quality life. Sometimes this is pure luck, but you can do much to keep the odds in your favor.

Take advantage of your convalescent period to review your priorities and to reflect on what risk factors led to your heart attack. Determine to make changes that will have lasting benefits.

Taking Low-Dose Aspirin

No matter what risk group you fall into, if you are not allergic you should take aspirin regularly to help prevent unwanted artery blood clots. This simple treatment has been shown to be very effective. (See pp. 45–46.)

Taking Fish Oil Supplements

You may want to consider taking a fish oil supplement, which can lower LDL cholesterol and support HDL cholesterol levels, as well as reducing the clotting tendency. (See p. 78.)

Using Beta Blocker Medications

Post-heart-attack patients are commonly prescribed a beta blocker (see p. 73) drug to take every day. This treatment is generally continued for up to a year, and can lower your chances of dying in that first year by 25 percent. If you have asthma, emphysema, heart failure, or, in some cases, diabetes, this treatment may not be suitable for you. As well, if you are in a very low risk group, you may not need a beta blocker after a heart attack.

If You Smoke

If you are a cigarette smoker who has survived a heart attack, smoking was an important reason for your illness. You must do all in your power to stop smoking. Your chances for sudden cardiac death are significantly reduced if you are able to discontinue this habit. As an ex-smoker you improve your chances of survival by 25 to 30 percent. (See *Detox* in SUGGESTED READING.)

Improving Your Cholesterol and Triglyceride Levels

If your cholesterol and triglyceride levels are abnormal, and especially if the ratio of your total cholesterol to HDL cholesterol is above the normal levels outlined in Chapter 3, your heart attack was at least partly caused by these imbalances. Resolve to do your best to correct these levels to improve your chances of long-term survival.

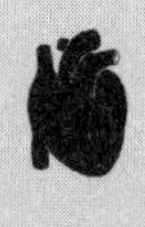

Improving your cholesterol and triglyceride levels will significantly boost your chances of long-term survival.

Set goals for yourself. Try for a few months to be disciplined about your diet and an exercise program. If your cholesterol levels do not show satisfactory improvement (see table below), your doctor may want you to consider taking medication.

Have your blood lipids (cholesterol and triglycerides) checked a few weeks after the heart attack rather than relying on tests done while you were in the hospital. The shock of the heart attack causes the readings done in that period to be out of kilter. Wait about 6 weeks after the heart attack to have your lipid levels checked.

Your post-heart-attack lipid goals:

Lipid	Goal
LDL Cholesterol	Below 130 mg/dL (3.36 mmol/L)
Triglycerides	Below 177 mg/dL (2.0 mmol/L)
HDL Cholesterol	Above 45 mg/dL (1.16 mmol/L)
Ratio of total/HDL cholesterol:	Below 4

If you are in an intermediate-risk or high-risk group, it may be a good idea to set more aggressive goals to try to reverse your coronary artery plaque:

Lipid	Goal
LDL Cholesterol	Below 100 mg/dL (2.6 mmol/L)
Triglycerides	Below 177 mg/dL (2.0 mmol/L)
HDL Cholesterol	Above 45 mg/dL (1.16 mmol/L)
Ratio of total/HDL cholesterol:	Below 3.5

Eating Foods Rich in L-Arginine or Taking Other Supplements

After a heart attack, it is particularly important to avoid magnesium depletion. Also, take the antioxidant vitamins C, E, and beta carotene, especially if their dietary sources are not prominent in your diet. (See p.82.)

Consider high doses of Vitamin B_{12} and folic acid. (See p. 49.)

If You Have High Blood Pressure

High blood pressure continues to be a dangerous risk factor after a heart attack. Keep your blood pressure in check through proper diet and exercise.

Your doctor may also prescribe medication. Effective blood pressure medications include members of the beta blocker family, preferably those that are "lipid neutral," such as acebutolol—that is, they do not worsen triglyceride and HDL cholesterol levels, as some beta blockers do. Another good choice for controlling high blood pressure in those with heart damage from previous heart attacks are members of the ACE inhibitor family. These cut down on the workload for each heartbeat and minimize the chances of future heart complications, such as heart failure. (See p. 72.)

High blood pressure should be lowered through diet, exercise, and, if necessary, medication.

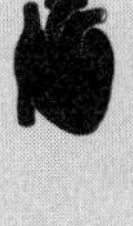

Getting Regular Exercise

Exercise will improve your sense of well-being, and lower your risk of unexpected cardiac death. You will need to have a professional exercise test, as described in Chapter 3, after your heart attack to give you guidelines for your exercise program. If possible, join a supervised exercise program designed for the post-heart-attack patient, such as those found at many community centers.

Sexual Activity

If you have had a heart attack, you and your partner may be concerned about resuming sexual activity. Medical research has established that sexual intercourse need not involve any more exertion than climbing a flight of stairs. If you can do this with relative comfort, you should have no heart problems with intercourse.

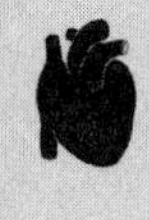

Sexual activity after a heart attack rarely poses a health risk.

Some men may become anxious about their potency. It is important for both you and your partner to be patient and understanding. If you experience persistent problems or anxiety, speak to your doctor about this. A counselling psychologist may be of help.

Maintaining a Positive Attitude

Do not isolate yourself. Many studies have shown that people who lack a social network are at much greater risk for heart attacks.

Try to foster a positive attitude and, above all, try not to feel sorry for yourself. Plan for the future rather than focusing on the past. But, if you are the sort of person who is inclined to deny that much is wrong with you, be careful not to overdo things for the first few months after your heart attack.

SUMMARY

- *Take control of your life by reviewing your priorities and making changes that will have lasting benefits for you.*
- *Take low-dose aspirin if suitable.*
- *Use prescribed beta blocker medications, if ordered by your doctor.*
- *If you are a smoker, overcome this habit.*
- *Know your cholesterol and triglyceride levels; keep them normal.*
- *Eat foods rich in L-arginine, or take supplements.*
- *Supplement your diet with antioxidants, suitable trace minerals, vitamins, and fish oil supplements.*
- *Maintain normal blood pressure.*
- *Exercise regularly.*
- *Resume sexual activity, keeping in mind that patience and understanding may be necessary.*
- *Maintain a positive attitude.*

About Medications and Treatments

9

CHOLESTEROL-LOWERING MEDICATIONS

Several medications that lower cholesterol levels are available. These include:

- *niacin (vitamin B_3)*
- *resins that bind bile acids*
- *fibric acid agents*
- *statins*

Cholesterol-lowering medications must be accompanied by lifestyle changes to be effective in the long term.

If your doctor has prescribed any of these medications to correct abnormalities in your cholesterol, you can expect dramatic improvement in your cholesterol levels.

Doctors frequently prescribe two medications from different families of cholesterol-lowering drugs—for example, niacin and a resin, or a statin and a resin. Certain combinations, however, should be used with caution.

Important Factors to Consider

Do not forget that medications for your cholesterol are secondary to your lifestyle changes. You should receive these medications only if your cholesterol levels need further improvement after changes of lifestyle and:

- *You have had a heart attack.*
- *You have angina.*
- *You have shown evidence of silent exertional ischemia. (See p. 6.)*
- *You have evidence of atherosclerosis in other areas, such as your lower extremities.*

When you receive a doctor's prescription, do not hesitate to ask such questions as:

- *How long should you take it?*
- *When should you return to determine its effects?*
- *What possible side effects might you experience?*

Niacin

This medication comes directly from nature. It is vitamin B_3, found in peanuts, poultry, fish, and green leafy plants. While large doses are required to treat cholesterol abnormalities, much improvement can be expected. It is an inexpensive medication.

Benefits

Niacin is especially beneficial for the total to HDL cholesterol ratio, since it increases HDL cholesterol while lowering LDL cholesterol. Niacin also lowers triglyceride levels.

Possible Side Effects

Although some people can use this drug for years without side effects, many people cannot tolerate the doses necessary to improve cholesterol levels. Possible side effects include:

- *unpleasant flushing*
- *skin rashes*
- *indigestion*
- *increased risk of getting gout, as niacin increases the blood uric acid level*
- *increased blood sugar level*

➠ *liver damage*

There is greatly increased risk of liver damage if you use sustained-release tablets. Avoid them.

If you take niacin, your blood must be checked periodically for increased levels of uric acid and blood sugar, and for liver function. Side effects can be minimized by splitting the dose, taking it with meals, and combining it with buffered aspirin (coated to prevent stomach upset). Since both aspirin and niacin are acids, their combined effect could irritate the stomach and result in stomach bleeding. The chance of this is lessened with buffered aspirin. The usefulness of aspirin is to cut down on uncomfortable flushing, but this effect tends to disappear after a few days or weeks. You can then reduce or discontinue the aspirin.

Always consult your doctor before taking medications, even those available without a prescription.

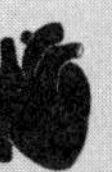

Dosage

To minimize side effects, you need to start with a quite low dose, 100 milligrams (mg) once or twice a day. Although many doctors eventually increase the dose to more than 3,000 mg per day to achieve the best possible cholesterol-lowering effect, a prudent dose may be 2,000 mg per day. The likelihood of side effects rises as the dose increases.

You can buy niacin over the counter. (Do not use sustained-release tablets.) But you should do so only with the advice and follow-up of your doctor. Avoid self-medication.

Resins

Two products containing bile acid resins are available by your doctor's prescription: cholestyramine and colestipol. They work by clinging to the cholesterol in bile that has been discharged from the liver into the small bowel. The polymer resin prevents the cholesterol from being reabsorbed, and carries it through into the feces.

Benefits

Resins that bind bile acids reduce elevated LDL cholesterol. They are compatible with niacin.

Possible Side Effects

Because the resins are not absorbed, their only side effects are related to the bowel: some bloating and indigestion may be experienced. If you are taking other medications, the resins may interfere with their absorption into the system. Therefore, other medications should be taken at a different time than the resin, such as first thing in the morning.

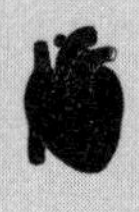

Resins prevent cholesterol from being reabsorbed into the body.

Dosage

Resins are powders that need to be mixed with food, such as applesauce or juice. They are packaged in individual doses or in a can with a scoop. They should be taken with meals, preferably the largest one.

Fibric Acid Agents

Several fibric acid agents are available by your doctor's prescription: clofibrate, gemfibrozil, fenofibrate, and others.

Benefits

These agents raise HDL cholesterol and decrease triglycerides. Your doctor may decide to combine fibric acid agents with resins; when used in combination, you will take lower doses of resins than when used alone.

Possible Side Effects

With each of the fibric acid agents, there is a slight chance of liver, blood, kidney, and muscular disorders. Your doctor can check for these with occasional blood and urine tests. Other side effects may include:

- *an increased chance of gallstones with clofibrate*
- *gaseousness*
- *indigestion*

Statins

The statins are a relatively new family of prescribed pharmaceuticals with powerful effects on blood cholesterol. Some generic names are lovastatin, simvastatin, and pravastatin.

Benefits

The statins usually cause a dramatic drop in LDL cholesterol of about 40 percent and a rise in HDL cholesterol of 5 to 10 percent. Thus, you can expect a significant improvement in your cholesterol ratio.

Long-term Side Effects of Statins

Thousands of patients have taken these medications over a period of years, with a low rate of side effects. While statins can be combined with resins, side effects could be more frequent if these drugs are taken with certain other medications, including fibric acid agents and high doses of niacin. Therefore, combining statins with these agents is reserved for difficult cases.

■ MEDICATIONS FOR HIGH BLOOD PRESSURE

If your blood pressure is high and does not respond to the nonmedicinal approaches already discussed, there are many choices of medication to lower blood pressure. Your doctor will choose one that seems to be suitable for you, but it is not uncommon to have to try different ones until you find the one (or combination) that is best for you.

You may need to try several medications for high blood pressure to find those most suitable for you.

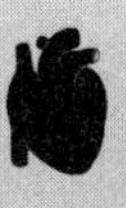

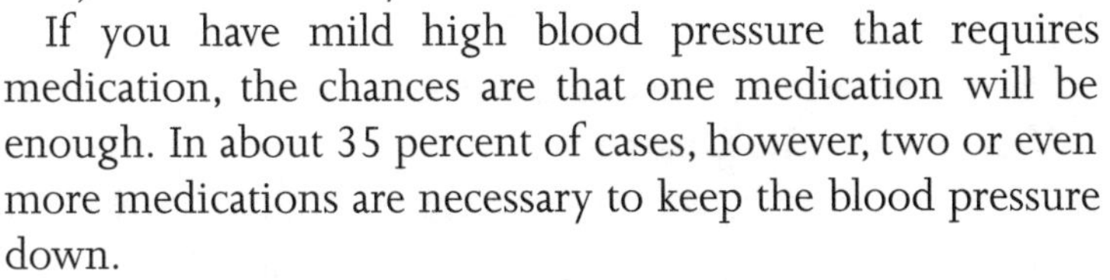

If you have mild high blood pressure that requires medication, the chances are that one medication will be enough. In about 35 percent of cases, however, two or even more medications are necessary to keep the blood pressure down.

Factors to Consider

To select the appropriate medication, your doctor will take the following factors into consideration:

- *cost. How much you can afford will need to be discussed. (But remember that many people spend a lot of money on cigarettes and liquor, which are not good for them. Spending an equivalent amount or less for control of blood pressure is a good investment.)*
- *your age*
- *whether or not you are athletic. Beta blockers, for example, cause your heart to be less efficient when you exercise strenuously.*
- *whether or not you have associated heart trouble, such as a previous heart attack or angina. Medications for blood pressure can be selected by your doctor to improve the coronary artery circulation, or spare the heart's energy.*
- *whether you have other conditions, such as asthma, emphysema, or diabetes. Beta blockers, for example, worsen asthma, and may mask symptoms of low blood sugar.*

No medication for high blood pressure is perfect. But remember that the advantages of preventing a heart attack or stroke far outweigh any of the minor disadvantages of having to take pills.

Types of Medications

There are three types of medications, all available with your doctor's prescription, to control high blood pressure:

1. Medications to expand your arteries so that your heart will encounter less resistance.
2. Medications to provide a smaller volume of blood within your circulation so that your heart needs to exert less pressure.
3. Medications to allow your heart to beat with less force so its pumping action is weakened.

Medications to Expand Arteries Via the Brain Center

These are centrally acting inhibitors of the sympathetic nervous system, but they are not commonly prescribed. Their generic names are methyldopa and clonidine.

Possible Side Effects
These are not common, and are generally mild and short term. They include drowsiness and dryness of the mouth.

Medications to Expand Arteries by Affecting Their Nerve Supply

The generic names of these medications are prazosin and terazosin.

Possible Side Effects
Although these medications are often useful, they need to be very carefully started. The first dose may cause an exaggerated drop in blood pressure, especially when you stand up. The result could be a fainting episode.
Your doctor will explain how to start these medications and the care you need to take. Other symptoms may be dizziness or headaches.

There are 3 approaches to lowering blood pressure with medications.

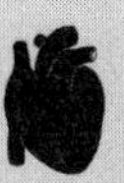

Medications to Expand the Arteries Directly

This family of medications, including hydralazine and loniten, is usually prescribed as a back-up treatment to reinforce the effect of another blood pressure pill. Loniten is reserved only for difficult and severe high blood pressure.

Possible Side Effects

- *fluid retention, causing swollen feet or possibly congested lungs, unless accompanied by a diuretic*
- *hair growth on the body and face (with loniten)*
- *palpitations due to more rapid heart rate*
- *flushing*
- *headaches*

Calcium Channel Blocker Medications That Expand the Arteries Indirectly

These medications block calcium from entering the muscle cells in the artery walls. The reduced amount of calcium in these cells causes the arteries to expand. Calcium channel blockers do not affect the stores of calcium in your bones or the calcium level in your blood. Their generic names are nifedipine, diltiazem, verapamil, nicardipine, and felodipine.

Possible Side Effects
These are infrequent but include:

- *headaches*
- *nausea or stomach upsets*
- *flushing*
- *swelling of feet*

ACE Inhibitors That Expand the Arteries Indirectly

Angiotensin converting enzyme (ACE) inhibitors block the formation of a powerful chemical that constricts arteries. This results in a lowering of blood pressure levels. Their generic names are captopril, enalopril, lisinopril, fosinopril, and quinapril.

Possible Side Effects
Many people take these pills without problems, but possible side effects include:

- *headaches*
- *dizziness*
- *fatigue*
- *skin rashes*
- *cough*

Medications to Reduce the Blood Volume

These pharmaceutical drugs are diuretics, which stimulate the kidneys to excrete salt and water. Some also get rid of potassium, which is not a desirable effect. Others not only get rid of salt and water, but actually conserve potassium. Their generic names are hydrochlorothiazide, furosemide, amiloride (potassium-retaining), spironolactone (potassium-retaining), and triamterene (potassium-retaining).

If you are on diuretic drugs, your doctor will want to check your blood sodium and potassium levels periodically.

Possible Side Effects

Side effects are uncommon but could include:

- *dryness of the mouth*
- *stomach or bowel upsets*
- *dizziness*

Diuretics help to reduce blood volume by forcing your body to excrete salt and water.

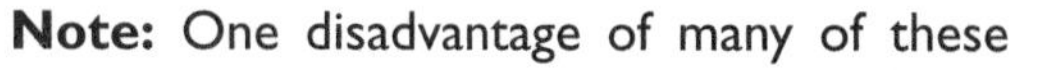

Note: One disadvantage of many of these drugs is that they can worsen your triglyceride and HDL cholesterol levels. Doctors are careful to give only light doses of these medications, and to monitor the lipid levels of their patients on diuretic therapy.

Beta Blocker Medications to Reduce the Force of the Heartbeat

These pharmaceutical medications reduce blood pressure in subtle ways that are still being researched. They cause the heart to beat more slowly and less forcefully by blocking the accelerator nerves to the heart muscle.

Beta blockers are commonly prescribed for those at high risk or who have had a heart attack.

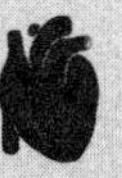

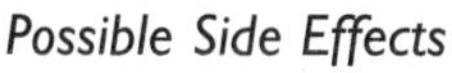

Possible Side Effects

Some of these drugs, especially if they are combined with a diuretic, will cause your triglyceride level to rise and your HDL level to decrease. Others (such as acebutolol and pindolol) are called "lipid-neutral" because they do not have this effect. Their generic names are acebutolol, atenolol, metoprolol, nadolol, pindolol, propranolol, and timolol.

ABOUT CHELATION THERAPY

Chelation therapy is still a controversial treatment for artery disease, although it has been used since the 1950s. A chelating agent, ethylene diamine tetra-acetic acid (EDTA), is given intravenously during a treatment lasting three to four

hours. EDTA binds with metals in the body, which are then excreted through the kidneys. An average course of chelation therapy involves 30 treatments.

Before a patient begins therapy and periodically during the course of treatment, blood tests will be done to check proper kidney functioning. Chelation therapy is considered safe when professionally administered.

Since researchers have found that many metals, including copper, iron, and lead, promote oxidation leading to artery disease, chelation treatments have been used to remove a variety of metals from the blood. While chelation therapy has been proven effective for removing metals, its value in regressing artery disease is questionable. (See *A Textbook on EDTA Chelation Therapy* in SUGGESTED READING.)

■ SUMMARY

A variety of medications for improving your lipids or your blood pressure, with the goal of heart attack prevention, is available by prescription from your doctor.

- *If your lipids put you at increased risk for heart attacks, yet there is no evidence of coronary (or other) atherosclerosis, rely entirely on lifestyle changes.*
- *If your lipid abnormalities are accompanied by coronary atherosclerosis, and do not respond adequately to lifestyle changes, you should discuss taking lipid-lowering drugs with your doctor.*
- *Niacin, a natural agent (Vitamin B_3) that is helpful for lipids, is available over the counter. But it is unwise to self-medicate yourself with niacin. Avoid sustained-release niacin.*
- *If your blood pressure remains high, despite appropriate lifestyle changes, there are a variety of blood pressure-lowering medications available by prescription that help to reduce your risk of both heart attacks and strokes.*
- *Since chelation therapy is unproven, do not abandon other treatments in favor of chelation.*

Daily Heart Attack Prevention Program

10

Adopting a healthy lifestyle will help you control your heart attack risk factors. This means eating properly, following an exercise program, and controlling your stress level.

If you are a smoker, quit, and if you live or work with smokers, do your utmost to avoid exposure to their smoke. (See p. 32–34.)

■ DAILY DIETARY STRATEGIES

In planning your daily menu, you must consider:

- *total calories*
- *total fat*
- *saturated fats*
- *unsaturated fats*
- *sugars and starches*
- *special proteins, L-arginine*
- *dietary cholesterol*
- *dietary fiber*
- *alcohol*
- *salt*
- *vitamins and minerals*
- *sufficient water*

Total Calories

If you are overweight, there is only one bottom line—your body is storing unused calories. To lose weight, you must take in fewer calories, burn more calories through exercise, and preferably both. Your HDL cholesterol will rise as you lose weight.

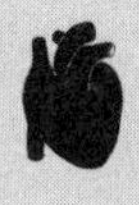

To lose weight, you must develop realistic goals and a program you can follow over time.

Ask your doctor for a sensible goal for your weight-loss program. Often this would be approximately what you weighed when you were 21. Ask your doctor or a nutritionist to help you develop a food plan to ensure that you consume the appropriate number and type of calories each day to reach and maintain that weight.

The following chart lists the number of calories per gram in various food sources.

Sources of Calories

Food Source	Calories per Ounce	Calories per Gram
Fat*	225	9.0
Alcohol	198**	7.0
Protein	113	4.0
Carbohydrate	113	4.0

* *Note that one ounce or gram of fat has twice the calories of the same amount of either protein or carbohydrate foods. Note also that alcohol has more calories per ounce or gram than carbohydrates and protein.*
** *See p. 45.*

Total Fat

To lose weight and lessen your chances of having a heart attack, reduce the fats in your diet to less than 30 percent of your total calories. Unless you are already being careful about your diet, its fat content is probably 36 percent or more. To reduce it to less than 30 percent, you must become aware of the sources of the fats you eat.

Most dietary fat comes from three sources:

1. *Margarines or oils, used for spreads, salad dressings, or cooking.*
2. *Meat, poultry, and fish.*
3. *Dairy foods: milk, cream, butter, cheese, yogurt, or ice cream.*

Watch also for the hidden fats contained in prepared products. For example, commercially baked goods contain hidden fats. Reduce your consumption of pies, cakes, doughnuts, croissants, muffins, biscuits, cookies, and crackers.

Saturated Fat

Saturated fats are the main culprits in driving up LDL cholesterol and aggravating the atherosclerotic process. These fats are derived mainly from animal sources, with two exceptions: coconut oil and palm oil. Since saturated fats stay solid at room temperature, in contrast to the liquid state of unsaturated vegetable fats, coconut or palm oil is often added to margarine and other spreads.

Read labels carefully to avoid the hidden fats in prepared foods.

Hydrogenated vegetable fats have been artifically saturated by the addition of hydrogen, in order to add more body. This process converts naturally occurring fatty acids into trans-fatty acids. These are not essential to body function. They raise LDL cholesterol levels, and promote atherosclerosis, significantly increasing heart attack risks. (See Chapter 14 for information on recent research.) Look for margarines or oils that are not hydrogenated, and avoid products containing hydrogenated oils (a common ingredient in commercially baked foods).

Unless you are carefully watching your diet, chances are that you are consuming far too much saturated fat. You should reduce your intake of saturated fat to less than 10 percent of your total calories. You can do this by cutting down on margarine and salad dressings, meats, dairy products, and bakery items. Appendices A and B list the percentage of total fat and saturated fat calories of various foods, and suggest some examples of foods to choose and to avoid. Use these tables to help you select foods that are low in total fat and saturated fats.

Saturated and hydrogenated fats raise LDL cholesterol levels and promote artery disease.

Unsaturated Fats

Although you can lower your total and LDL cholesterol by consuming unsaturated fats, you should take these in strict moderation. Vegetable fats are mostly unsaturated, but all contain some saturated fat. Exceptions are coconut and palm oils, which are heavily saturated.

Polyunsaturated Fats

Unsaturated fats may be polyunsaturated or monounsaturated. Polyunsaturated fats may belong to either the omega 3 or the omega 6 family. Omega 6 fats lower both your HDL cholesterol and your LDL cholesterol, but omega 3 fats help support levels of HDL cholesterol while lowering your LDL cholesterol. This means that your ratio of total to HDL cholesterol decreases to more desirable levels with omega 3 fats, but not with omega 6 fats.

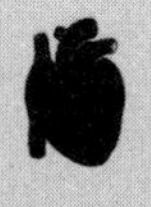

Omega 3 fats raise HDL (good) cholesterol and lower LDL (bad) cholesterol levels.

Omega 3 fats have special qualities beneficial for the long-term goal of heart attack prevention. The most desirable omega 3 fat is eicosapentoic acid (EPA), found mainly in certain fish. The average North American diet is low in omega 3 fats, and heavy in omega 6 fats (found in vegetable and nut oils). (See APPENDIX C for the omega 3 content of various fish species.)

You may prefer to augment your diet with concentrated fish oil supplements, containing up to 1,000 mg or more of EPA per day. These are available from health stores. If you do, remember that each capsule contains at least 10 calories and about 5 milligrams of cholesterol. Nevertheless, the benefits of regular consumption of fish oil concentrate outweigh the small amount of cholesterol it adds to your diet. When choosing your supplements, check the label for the strength of EPA in each capsule.

Note: Try to find out if the fish you buy comes from a safe source, to minimize your ingestion of mercury and other pollutants. Do not eat fish livers or other organs. Some commercial fish oil supplements are screened for contaminants, and are pollutant-free. This may not be marked on the label, so ask your supplier for this information.

Monounsaturated Fats:
Monounsaturated fatty acids also promote heart health. The important monounsaturated fatty acid in nutrition is oleic acid (the omega 9 family), which is the main ingredient in olive oil. Below are some suggested choices for cooking or salad oils:

- *canola oil*
- *olive oil*
- *almond oil*
- *pistachio oil*
- *pumpkin oil*
- *sesame oil*
- *safflower oil*
- *sunflower oil*
- *corn oil*
- *walnut oil*
- *peanut oil*

Sugars and Starches

Carbohydrates may be either simple (sugars) or complex (starches). Dieting successfully to lose weight means reducing the fat and sugar content of your diet in favor of starch. Common sources of starches are breads, cereals, pastas, legumes, vegetables, and fruits.

To reduce your intake of sugar, learn to enjoy sugarless coffee, tea, and cereals.

Special Proteins

Choose soybean products. The protein in soybean has special cholesterol-lowering effects. Tofu (soybean curd) is rich in this substance.

Also, eat suitable quantities of seeds, nuts, and legumes rich in the amino acid L-arginine. (See pp. 41 and 138.)

Dietary Cholesterol

Most of the cholesterol you take in with your food is expelled through your bowel. However, we vary in how our bodies handle food cholesterol. If you have coronary artery disease, or a high cholesterol from an inherited disorder (familial hypercholesterolemia), strictly limit the cholesterol in your food.

How your dietary cholesterol will affect your blood cholesterol level is closely tied to the amount of saturated fat you are consuming. If you eat a diet high in saturated fat, the cholesterol in your food will more readily raise your blood cholesterol. But, if you keep to a low-saturated-fat (and high-fiber) diet, mild to moderate amounts of cholesterol in your diet usually have either no effect or only a minor effect on your blood cholesterol.

If you are not at high risk of a heart attack, a small amount of cholesterol in your diet will not significantly raise your cholesterol levels.

Egg yolk is the main cholesterol-rich food in our diet. So if you want to lower your blood cholesterol, the usual advice is to eliminate egg yolks from your diet. This is good advice if you have familial hypercholesterolemia or if your heart attack risk is great, and you are on a program aimed at reversing the cholesterol-laden plaques. But if your risks of a heart attack are only moderate, and if you are following a low-fat, high-fiber diet, three or four eggs per week will not affect your blood cholesterol.

Dietary Fiber

Fiber, especially water-soluble fiber, helps improve your cholesterol levels and your blood pressure. Cholesterol attaches to the fiber and is excreted through the bowel.

The best sources of fiber are grains, fruits, and vegetables. Animal products contain no fiber. To ensure that you get adequate fiber in your diet, follow these guidelines:

- *Choose whole fruits over fruit juices.*
- *Choose oat cereals or other oat products over wheat products. (Oats are water soluble.)*

- *Chick peas and other legumes can lower your cholesterol.*
- *Guar gum, a gummy fiber from certain beans, is an effective cholesterol-lowering fiber.*

Dietary fiber helps to lower both cholesterol and blood pressure levels.

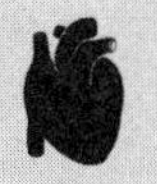

Many foods that are high in fiber contain pectin, which also lowers cholesterol. Common sources of pectin and their relative pectin content are as follows: high—figs, oranges, pears, potatoes; intermediate—sweet potatoes, soybeans, Brussels sprouts, apples, lima beans; lower—carrots, papaya, peanuts.

Alcohol

If you cannot moderate your intake of alcohol, you need to avoid it completely. Otherwise, the moderate use of alcohol, whether beer, wine, or spirits, can help to protect you from heart attacks, as it helps prevent blood clots. Red wine contains potent antioxidants. (See page 82.) The following chart gives maximum daily guidelines for alcohol consumption. Most people will prefer smaller amounts. Avoid binge drinking.

Maximum Daily Intake of Alcohol

Drink	Ounces
Beer	24
Wine	8
Whiskey, gin, etc.	2

Salt

Restrict your salt intake if you have high blood pressure. But even if you are under 60 and your blood pressure is normal, it is still wise to restrict your salt intake to prevent the blood pressure increases that are more common after 60.

Some tips for reducing salt in your diet:

- *Ban the salt shaker from your table, and don't add salt when cooking.*

- *Avoid processed meats, such as sausages, bacon, and smoked deli meats.*
- *Avoid commercial soups and prepared foods—unless labelled "low salt."*
- *Use garlic, onions, ginger, herbs, lemon juice, vinegar, and pepper as replacements for salt. These food items may help improve your cholesterol levels as well as reduce the chances of unwanted blood clots.*

Vitamins and Trace Minerals

Mild to moderate vitamin and trace mineral deficiencies are common, and correcting them is important in heart attack prevention. In recent years, there have been encouraging studies on the significance of vitamins and minerals to heart health. (See Chapter 14.) If you are at risk of a heart attack, you should use supplements. Appendix D lists the benefits of selected vitamins and minerals, common food sources, and suggested daily supplements. Your physician or dietitian may recommend higher doses.

Antioxidants

Antioxidants, whether they come from vitamin- and mineral-rich foods or from supplements, help to protect you from the destructive effects of an inner process called peroxidation. Among its other bad effects is the hastening of atherosclerosis. The artery disease is partially caused by the oxidation of LDL cholesterol.

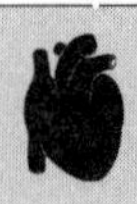

Antioxidants help to protect against artery disease.

Among the antioxidant vitamins are beta carotene (pro-vitamin A), and vitamins C and E. The mineral selenium is an antioxidant, and helps fight the harmful effects of copper. (See below.) HDL cholesterol is also considered to have antioxidant properties.

Vitamin C is now considered particularly important in the prevention of heart disease, so include vitamin C supplements containing at least 500 mg, and preferably 1,000 mg, to your daily diet (but see iron, below).

Copper and Iron

Copper and iron are potent promoters of peroxidation and excess levels have been associated with an increased risk of heart attacks. Fortunately, copper excess is not common. If you live in a "soft" water area, there is an increased risk of copper in the drinking water, especially when copper pipes are used for plumbing. Levels of both copper and iron (as ferritin) can be tested in blood samples. (See About Chelation Therapy, pp. 73–74.)

Note: If you are already at risk for heart attack, and unless you are subject to iron deficiency anemia, do not take vitamin or mineral supplements containing iron. Additionally, megadoses of vitamin C may aggravate heart attack risk by enhancing iron overload, if you are genetically vulnerable. Checking your serum ferritin level will show if your iron stores are excessive.

Drinking Water

Your drinking water influences your heart attack risk, especially in respect to sudden cardiac death.

"Hard" water areas have a lower rate of sudden cardiac death than "soft" water communities. The main hard water mineral is calcium, together with magnesium, zinc, and selenium. There is no clear link that indicates which one (or ones) affords the protection. However, patients dying of heart disease often have lower than normal levels of magnesium. Doctors have used magnesium to combat rhythm disorders.

If you are a heart patient living in a soft water community, ask your doctor about safe mineral supplements, and about the possibility of excess copper. (See above.)

■ EXERCISE FOR HEART ATTACK PREVENTION

Lack of exercise is a major risk factor for heart attacks. Exercise improves your blood pressure, helps combat obesity and improves your HDL cholesterol and your ratio of total cholesterol to HDL cholesterol. You are less likely to suffer sudden cardiac death if you exercise regularly. Exercising is also an effective way to reduce stress.

Before You Start

If you have any risk factors for heart attacks, ask your doctor if you need a professional exercise test to determine the limits of safe exercise for you. (If you are not in the age group where heart attacks are likely, this may not be necessary.) After such a test, your doctor can give you guidelines for a heart rate that is safe for you, and tell you what rate you should not exceed.

Your Safe Heart Rate

To find your heart rate, check your pulse immediately after stopping exercise. Count your pulse for 10 seconds, and multiply the rate by 6 to get the total number of beats per minute.

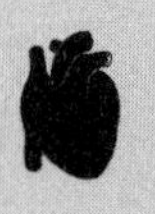

If you have not been physically active, ask your doctor for help in developing a safe exercise program.

Find your pulse either at your wrist, or preferably in the neck. In the neck, press firmly inward just under your jaw bone where it connects with an imaginary line from the bottom of your ear.

First practice checking your pulse rate when you are at rest, then learn to do it after exercise.

Choosing an Exercise Program to Suit You

The type of exercise program you choose must fulfill the following requirements:

- *It must be safe for you.*

  If you have any risk factors for heart attacks, first find out from your doctor how much you can exert yourself, and what heart rate you should aim for. If you have heart trouble, consider attending supervised exercise classes at your local community center or fitness center.

  If you choose brisk walking or running, you need to do it in a safe location. Icy streets and heavy traffic can be both unhealthy and dangerous. Be cautious, to avoid muscular and joint (including back) strains.

➠ *It must be simple.*

Choosing a simple form of exercise increases your chances of sticking with it. Walking, jogging, and running are good choices because they are uncomplicated. No equipment is required—just good shoes and loose, comfortable clothing. Moreover, you can walk, jog, or run any time it suits you. Walking causes less physical strain than running.

Your exercise program must be safe, simple, aerobic, regular, and fun.

Dancing may be more complicated if you want to enroll in a class or go to a dance club. Depending on the type of dance you like, you may need a partner. Nevertheless, many people continue this activity for years.

Swimming is excellent exercise, but you need access to a pool, and the hours you can use it will, of course, be restricted.

Aerobic classes are popular and effective. No special equipment or clothing is required— except good shoes and loose, comfortable clothing—but you do have to be able to get to the classes at a designated time.

➠ *It must be moderately energetic.*

Choose a form of exercise that is aerobic: your heart needs to have a workout. The type of exercise you choose should provide rhythmic activity of the extremities, preferably the lower extremities. Fast walking, jogging, running, dancing, and swimming are all forms of aerobic exercise.

Your heart rate should rise to a suitable level for your age and your tolerance. If your doctor has indicated no limitations, try to achieve a heart rate of over 130 beats per minute, and maintain this rate for several minutes.

If you are not puffing, your workout is too easy. But if you become uncomfortable, slow down, get your breath, and then gradually speed up again.

Avoid shallow breathing. Find a harmony between your breathing and your body movements. Your heart will find its rhythm accordingly. (Weight training is not aerobic exercise, and is unsuitable for the aim of heart attack prevention.)

- *It should be uninterrupted.*

  The exercise should be steady and last at least 20 minutes. Find a good rhythm.
- *It should be done on a regular basis.*

  Exercise no less than three times a week to maintain your conditioning. Don't wait for the mood to strike. You need to pre-arrange your schedule. Choose the most suitable time of day and stick to it.
- *It should be enjoyable.*

  You are not likely to maintain a habit you do not enjoy. If you decide to exercise with a group, do your best to develop a camaraderie. If you are on your own, find a pleasant environment. Combining two types of exercise may be better for you—for example, jogging on your own once or twice a week, and going to an aerobics class the other times.

A Few Hints For Exercising

- *Warm up before you begin exercising. Gradually work up to your maximum intensity.*
- *Respect your body. Do not overexert. On the other hand, don't baby yourself. Be your own stern coach!*
- *Cool down after heavy exertion by walking and stretching for a few minutes.*
- *Drink fluids to replace those lost through perspiration.*

Special Precautions

Combined Altitude, Cold, and Exertion

Do not overexert yourself in extremely hot or cold weather, or at very high altitudes.

If your risk for a heart attack is quite strong and you are a skier, be very cautious about the triad of altitude, cold, and exertion. The altitude causes less oxygen to be available; breathing cold air causes the blood pressure to rise, the heart to accelerate, and the coronary arteries to constrict; the effort of skiing causes the heart to need more oxygen and blood.

Skiers at risk for heart attacks would be wise to choose spring-like conditions for their sport, and to be guided by their medical advisors about the amount of exertion that is safe.

Exertion in the Cold or Heat

Anyone at risk for a heart attack should avoid strenuous exertion in very cold or extremely hot conditions. Find an indoor location for your aerobic activities in the winter. In the summer, enjoy your exercise early, or late in the day.

■ LOWER YOUR STRESS LEVEL

Studies have shown that people who are overstressed are at a much higher risk of heart attacks. Here are some strategies for controlling stress.

- *Get away.*

  Stress becomes troublesome when it causes you to feel trapped. If you can get away for a few minutes, hours, or days, you can reduce the bad effects of stress. If you cannot get away physically, train your mind to transport you, even if only for a few minutes, out of the stressful situation. One way is to recall a delightful and relaxing experience in your past.

- *Exercise regularly.*

  To reduce stress this should be rhythmic, and involve the larger muscles, preferably the legs. Walking is a good choice. It has the advantage of temporarily getting you away from your responsibilities, and it unlocks stressed muscles.

- *Avoid monotony.*

  Monotony is a powerful producer of stress. Give yourself different tasks. Make a change. A hobby can be invaluable for stress relief.

Managing and reducing stress are vital for a healthy heart.

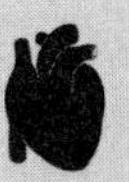

- *Try relaxation techniques.*

  Yoga, meditation, oriental breathing practices, and other relaxation techniques can relieve stress. You may want to listen to soothing music or the sounds of nature while you do these techniques.

- *Take time for yourself every day.*

  Enjoy some privacy.

- *Socialize with friends regularly.*

  Visit friends, invite them over for tea, or call them on the phone. Socializing need not be a big event, but feeling connected to other people can go a long way toward alleviating stress.

- *Talk about things that bother you.*

  Being able to talk over your problems with a person you trust helps to relieve stress. Heart attacks have been found to be more common in people who are lonely and isolated. Support groups help to reduce this risk.

Travel

Travelling on a commercial flight is quite safe if you are at risk for a heart attack, unless your symptoms are quite severe. If you can climb ten or twelve steps without symptoms, you should be able to fly without problems.

The stress of travel can cause as many (or more) heart attacks in the airport than in the plane. Heart attacks during flights are rare. Most occur in middle-aged men who had no history of heart trouble.

Travelling to high altitude locations is generally safe, unless your heart trouble is quite advanced. You can expect your heart rate to increase somewhat, but your blood pressure should change very little, if you go from sea level to 5,000 or more feet of altitude.

SUMMARY

Your daily guidelines for preventing a heart attack include learning to enjoy heart-healthy foods, taking sensible supplements, being conservative with alcohol, exercising regularly and safely, practicing effective stress-reducing measures, and not smoking.

A Chart For Your Progress Toward Heart Health

II

To achieve long-term heart attack prevention, you must make changes in your lifestyle, and make those new habits a permanent part of the way you live.

■ YOUR PROGRESS CHART

Using the Progress Chart will help you:

- *Compare your risk factor results over a period of time.*
- *Make both short-term and long-term goals.*
- *Observe the effect of dietary discipline, exercise, and medication on your risk factors.*

How to Fill in the Chart

- *Use Chart 1 if your test results are measured in mg/dL, or use Chart 3 if they are in mmol/L.*
- *In the first box under "Dates," write the month and year (e.g. 10/94) for which you are recording data. You may fill in the chart every few months, according to your doctor's advice.*
- *Fill in your total cholesterol, HDL cholesterol, LDL cholesterol, triglycerides, and the ratio of total cholesterol to HDL cholesterol for that date. You can get these figures from your doctor.*
- *Fill in your current weight.*

- *In the space for dietary discipline, rate that factor on a scale of 1 to 4 according to the following criteria:*
  1. *You have paid no attention to your diet.*
  2. *You have been only mildly self-disciplined in following your diet.*
  3. *You have been moderately self-disciplined in following your diet.*
  4. *You are adhering very strictly to your diet.*

  For more accuracy, you may wish to use a scale of 1, 1+, 2, 2+, 3, 3+, 4, 4+ for this and the following scales.
- *Rate your physical exercise habits on a scale of 1 to 4 according to the following criteria:*
  1. *You have been mostly sedentary.*
  2. *You have been mildly active.*
  3. *You have been moderately active.*
  4. *You have adhered strictly to a strenuous exercise program.*
- *Enter your blood pressure reading. If you have had more than one reading during the time period, use the average level.*
- *Indicate the average number of cigarettes you have smoked per day in the appropriate space.*
- *Rate how you have managed stress on a scale of 1 to 4 according to the following criteria:*
  1. *You have managed stress poorly.*
  2. *You have occasionally managed stress well.*
  3. *You have frequently but not always managed stress well.*
  4. *You consistently manage stress well.*
- *List the medications and supplements you are taking. Put the letter S in the appropriate date column to show when you start a medication. Use the letter C in subsequent months to show you are continuing the medication. Use the letter D to show when you discontinue it.*
- *The fourth page of each chart is reserved for your goals. In the extreme right-hand column are examples of ideal goals for your*

lipids, but these may need to be adjusted by your doctor. If you have angina or have had a heart attack, you may be advised to aim for even lower total cholesterol levels, lower LDL cholesterol levels, and lower total cholesterol to HDL cholesterol ratios than those shown. You should also fill in the weight you eventually wish to achieve, your goals for dietary discipline and physical exercise, your ideal blood pressure, and so on.

Be sure to fill in your Progress Chart completely and at regular intervals to get the most benefit from its use.

- *For short-term goals, list your objectives for the next few months. For example, by 12/94 you may wish to lower your cholesterol levels to a certain degree, to weigh 5 pounds less, and to increase your dietary discipline from 1 to 3.*

AN EXAMPLE OF A PATIENT WITH ANGINA

Charts 2 and 4 show how a patient suffering from the recent onset of angina used a progress chart between February 1990 and June 1992. Her condition was quite serious, and she would therefore have been examined more frequently by her doctor than the average patient.

She quit smoking (20 cigarettes a day) in February 1990. At the same time, she adopted a new diet that was low in fats and cholesterol, and high in fiber. Her dietary discipline improved from 1 in February 1990 to 3 in May, causing a modest drop in her total cholesterol, her triglycerides, and the ratio of total cholesterol to HDL cholesterol.

With the aim of shrinking the plaque, she began taking niacin while continuing with her strict dietary regime. When her lipids were rechecked in September, her HDL cholesterol had risen well, and her LDL cholesterol was slightly reduced. The dose of niacin was then increased, and cholestyramine (a resin to reduce blood cholesterol) was added to augment the effects of niacin. Later she developed a skin rash and therefore stopped taking niacin. She was started on lovastatin (another drug to reduce cholesterol) in April 1991, and thereafter continued with this medication and the cholestyramine.

PROGRESS CHART No. 1 (U.S. Units—mg/dL)				
ITEMS	**DATES**			
Total Cholesterol				
HDL Cholesterol				
LDL Cholesterol				
Triglycerides				
Ratio of Total Chol./HDL Chol.				
Weight (lbs.)				
Dietary Discipline*				
Physical Exercise**				
Blood Pressure				
Cigarettes/Day				
Stress Management†				
Medications & Supplements††				

PROGRESS CHART No. 1 cont. (U.S. Units—mg/dL)					
DATES					

PROGRESS CHART No. 1 cont. (U.S. Units—mg/dL)				
ITEMS	DATES			
Total Cholesterol				
HDL Cholesterol				
LDL Cholesterol				
Triglycerides				
Ratio of Total Chol./HDL Chol.				
Weight (lbs.)				
Dietary Discipline*				
Physical Exercise**				
Blood Pressure				
Cigarettes/Day				
Stress Management†				
Medications & Supplements††				

PROGRESS CHART No. 1 cont. (U.S. Units—mg/dL)

OBJECTIVES					
SHORT TERM			LONG TERM		
					< 200
					> 45
					< 130
					< 150
					< 4.5

*Dietary Discipline: 1 (Undisciplined) to 4 (Most Disciplined)
**Physical Exercise: 1 (Least Active) to 4 (Most Active)
†Stress Management: 1 (Poor) to 4 (Most Favorable)
††Medications & Supplements:
S = Start; D = Discontinue; C = Continue

SAMPLE PROGRESS CHART No. 2 (U.S. Units—mg/dL)				
Name: Mrs. E.M.		**Date of Birth: Dec. 28/22**		
ITEMS	**DATES**			
	02/90	**05/90**	**09/90**	**12/90**
Total Cholesterol	317	287	292	238
HDL Cholesterol	57	56	63	66
LDL Cholesterol		197	195	134
Triglycerides	216	174	169	191
Ratio of Total Chol./HDL Chol.	5.6	5.2	4.6	3.6
Weight (lbs.)	125	127	130	127
Dietary Discipline*	1	3	3	4
Physical Exercise**	2	2	2	2
Blood Pressure	140/80	110/70	130/70	
Cigarettes/Day	20	0	0	0
Stress Management†	3	3	3	3
Medications & Supplements††				
Niacin		S	C	C
Cholestyramine			S	C
Lovastatin				
Aspirin	S	C	C	C
Premarin (estrogen)				
Vitamins C & E		S	C	C
Beta Carotene				

SAMPLE CHART No. 2 cont. (U.S. Units—mg/dL)

DATES					
04/91	**08/91**	**12/91**	**06/92**		
284	225	206	212		
58	59		60		
154	119		120		
354	234		164		
4.9	3.8		3.6		
128	126		125		
4	4	4	4		
2	3	2+	2+		
110/70	110/70	110/70	110/70		
0	0	0	0		
3	3	3	4		
S					
C	C	C	C		
S	C	C	C		
C	C	C	C		
		S	C		
C	C	C	C		
	S	C	C		

SAMPLE CHART No. 2 cont. (U.S. Units—mg/dL)				
ITEMS	**DATES**			
Total Cholesterol				
HDL Cholesterol				
LDL Cholesterol				
Triglycerides				
Ratio of Total Chol./HDL Chol.				
Weight (lbs.)				
Dietary Discipline*				
Physical Exercise**				
Blood Pressure				
Cigarettes/Day				
Stress Management†				
Medications & Supplements††				

SAMPLE CHART No. 2 cont. (U.S. Units—mg/dL)

OBJECTIVES					
SHORT TERM			LONG TERM		
04/90	04/91	08/91	06/92		
253	219	241	213		< 200
58	58	59	60		> 45
		134	120		< 100
< 200	< 200	< 200	< 200		< 150
4.4	3.8	4.1	3.5		< 4.5
	127	127	127		125
4	4	4	4		4
2+	2+	2+	2+		3
110/70	110/70	110/70	110/70		110/70
0	0	0	0		0
4	4	4	4		4

*Dietary Discipline: 1 (Undisciplined) to 4 (Most Disciplined)

**Physical Exercise: 1 (Least Active) to 4 (Most Active)

†Stress Management: 1 (Poor) to 4 (Most Favorable)

††Medications & Supplements:
S = Start; D = Discontinue; C = Continue

PROGRESS CHART No. 3 (Int'l Units—mmol/dL)				
ITEMS	**DATES**			
Total Cholesterol				
HDL Cholesterol				
LDL Cholesterol				
Triglycerides				
Ratio of Total Chol./HDL Chol.				
Weight (lbs.)				
Dietary Discipline*				
Physical Exercise**				
Blood Pressure				
Cigarettes/Day				
Stress Management†				
Medications & Supplements††				

PROGRESS CHART No. 3 cont. (Int'l Units—mmol/dL)					
DATES					

PROGRESS CHART No. 3 cont. (Int'l Units—mmol/dL)				
ITEMS	**DATES**			
Total Cholesterol				
HDL Cholesterol				
LDL Cholesterol				
Triglycerides				
Ratio of Total Chol./HDL Chol.				
Weight (lbs.)				
Dietary Discipline*				
Physical Exercise**				
Blood Pressure				
Cigarettes/Day				
Stress Management†				
Medications & Supplements††				

PROGRESS CHART No. 3 cont. (Int'l Units—mmol/dL)

OBJECTIVES					
SHORT TERM			LONG TERM		
					< 5.16
					< 1.16
					< 3.40
					< 1.69
					< 4.5

*Dietary Discipline: 1 (Undisciplined) to 4 (Most Disciplined)
**Physical Exercise: 1 (Least Active) to 4 (Most Active)
†Stress Management: 1 (Poor) to 4 (Most Favorable)
††Medications & Supplements:
S = Start; D = Discontinue; C = Continue

SAMPLE PROGRESS CHART No. 4 (Int'l Units—mmol/dL)				
Name: Mrs. E.M.		**Date of Birth: Dec. 28/22**		
ITEMS	**DATES**			
	02/90	**05/90**	**09/90**	**12/90**
Total Cholesterol	8.18	7.43	7.55	6.14
HDL Cholesterol	1.47	1.44	1.63	1.70
LDL Cholesterol		5.09	5.05	3.46
Triglycerides	2.44	1.97	1.91	2.16
Ratio of Total Chol./HDL Chol.	5.6	5.2	4.6	3.6
Weight (lbs.)	125	127	130	127
Dietary Discipline*	1	3	3	4
Physical Exercise**	2	2	2	2
Blood Pressure	140/80	110/70	130/70	
Cigarettes/Day	20	0	0	0
Stress Management†	3	3	3	3
Medications & Supplements††				
Niacin		S	C	C
Cholestyramine			S	C
Lovastatin				
Aspirin	S	C	C	C
Premarin (estrogen)				
Vitamins C & E		S	C	C
Beta Carotene				

SAMPLE CHART No. 4 cont. (Int'l Units—mmol/dL)					
DATES					
04/91	**08/91**	**12/91**	**06/92**		
7.34	5.81	5.33	5.47		
1.51	1.53		1.54		
3.97	3.08		3.09		
4.0	2.65		1.85		
4.9	3.8		3.6		
128	126		125		
4	4	4	4		
2	3	2+	2+		
110/70	110/70	110/70	110/70		
0	0	0	0		
3	3	3	4		
S					
C	C	C	C		
S	C	C	C		
C	C	C	C		
		S	C		
C	C	C	C		
	S	C	C		

SAMPLE CHART No. 4 cont. (Int'l Units—mmol/dL)

ITEMS	DATES			
Total Cholesterol				
HDL Cholesterol				
LDL Cholesterol				
Triglycerides				
Ratio of Total Chol./HDL Chol.				
Weight (lbs.)				
Dietary Discipline*				
Physical Exercise**				
Blood Pressure				
Cigarettes/Day				
Stress Management†				
Medications & Supplements††				

SAMPLE CHART No. 4 cont. (Int'l Units—mmol/dL)					
OBJECTIVES					
SHORT TERM			**LONG TERM**		
04/90	**04/91**	**08/91**	**06/92**		
6.54	5.65	6.23	5.5		< 5.16
1.49	1.50	1.52	1.55		< 1.16
		3.45	1.9		< 2.60
< 2.0	< 2.0	< 2.0	< 2.0		< 1.69
4.4	3.8	4.1	3.5		< 4.0
	127	127	127		125
4	4	4	4		4
2+	2+	2+	2+		3
110/70	110/70	110/70	110/70		110/70
0	0	0	0		0
4	4	4	4		4

*Dietary Discipline: 1 (Undisciplined) to 4 (Most Disciplined)

**Physical Exercise: 1 (Least Active) to 4 (Most Active)

†Stress Management: 1 (Poor) to 4 (Most Favorable)

††Medications & Supplements:
S = Start; D = Discontinue; C = Continue

■ SUMMARY

The Progress Chart can help you and your doctor keep track of your long-term progress with heart attack prevention goals. You can see the effects of your behavior changes—especially changes in your dietary discipline and exercise habits—on your weight and other risk factors. When you can see the progress you have made, you will be better motivated to keep up your healthy lifestyle over the long term.

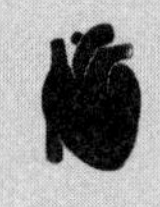

Your doctor may want to adjust the figures suggested for long-term objectives.

Symptoms Mistaken for a Heart Attack

12

Several conditions that are not related to heart disease can make you think you are about to have a heart attack. A description of some of these conditions and their symptoms follows. However, do not diagnose yourself. This information is for your general knowledge only. Your doctor will make the diagnosis.

CONDITIONS THAT MAY MIMIC HEART ATTACK SYMPTOMS

Pericarditis

Pericarditis is an inflammation of the outer lining of the heart that is not at all related to coronary heart disease. The chest pain, though, is similar to the pain you might feel if you were having a heart attack. The pain is usually steady, and is aggravated by deep breathing and by lying down.

Pericarditis is usually accompanied by a fever. Most often it is caused by a virus, but there are numerous other possible causes, including tuberculosis, cancer, systemic lupus erythematosis, or a recent heart attack.

Paroxysmal Atrial Tachycardia (PAT)

You may be well and fit but suddenly feel a pounding of your heart that makes you feel anxious. Your heart rate has suddenly jumped from its usual rate of about 70 beats per minute to anywhere from 140 to 220 beats per minute. This usually occurs in people in their 20s or 30s. It is not a heart attack but paroxysmal atrial tachycardia, related to the special tissue that transmits electric impulses throughout the heart. It may last a few seconds, or occasionally, hours. In most cases, your heart will rein itself in from its wild gallop to a walking pace.

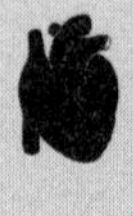

PAT most often affects young adults, and usually stops without medical assistance.

Paroxysmal Atrial Fibrillation

If you are middle-aged or older, and you have symptoms that are similar to those of PAT, they are likely to be due to paroxysmal atrial fibrillation. With this condition, your heart beats quickly but irregularly. Although some victims have a background of coronary atherosclerosis, for many people the rhythm disturbance is an isolated condition.

Valvular Heart Disease (VHD)

You may have shortness of breath when you walk, and other symptoms that are typical of angina. (See pp. 6–7.) But if you have valvular heart disease, your symptoms are due not to coronary atherosclerosis but to faulty heart valves.

Although your heart has four valves, only two are commonly affected by VHD—the mitral valve or the aortic valve. Most cases of VHD used to be caused by rheumatic fever. Now that rheumatic fever is rare in North America, you are more likely to have a leaky mitral valve or a tight (stenosed) aortic valve as a result of degenerative changes in the valves. In the case of a leaky mitral valve, the valve tissue is too floppy. If VHD is very severe, you may need valve replacement surgery.

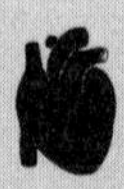

Valvular heart disease can mimic angina symptoms.

Cardiomyopathy

This condition is relatively uncommon but can be serious. It is a disease of the heart muscle, often without a known cause. If you have cardiomyopathy, your heart muscle is weak and you are subject to eventual heart failure. In most cases, the coronary arteries are quite normal. Prescribed medications can reduce symptoms and improve your lifespan.

Vaso-Vagal Syncope

This is the medical term for a simple faint. If you have an unexpected fainting spell, you or your friends may worry about your heart.

Fainting is rarely linked to heart problems.

If the fainting spell occurs when you are upset about seeing something unpleasant, such as a car accident, or when you have been standing too long in a hot room, the diagnosis of vaso-vagal syncope is not difficult. But if it occurs when you would not expect it, you may need to see a doctor to have other possibilities, such as an atypical heart attack, ruled out.

Asthma or Emphysema

If you have bronchial asthma or lung disease you will feel short of breath and experience a tightness in the chest. These symptoms are similar to those of angina. If you have either asthma or emphysema *and* angina, it may be difficult for you and your doctor to separate the symptoms of the bronchial condition from those of the cardiac condition. The exercise electrocardiogram or other tests mentioned in Chapter 3 will help to show which condition is primarily responsible for your symptoms.

Hyperventilation

If you have a suffocating discomfort and feel you cannot take a deep enough breath, it is not necessarily your heart. It may be that your chest wall muscles and diaphragm are tightening up as a result of stress. This is known as hyperventilation. Even if you have coronary disease and angina, hyperventilation may add to your symptoms.

Hyperventilation is an acute reaction to stress, but is not itself life-threatening.

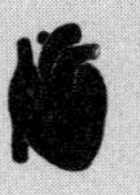

If you have a severe spell of hyperventilation, you will feel panicky, which aggravates the whole situation. You feel out of control and weak, and may experience numbness and tingling of the lips and hands.

Although this is a terrifying experience, it is not at all life-threatening. Being aware of what is happening in the early moments of an episode will help you to avoid the panic stage.

Stress-reducing practices (see pp. 87–88) will help to prevent these occurrences.

Anemia

If you are anemic and you have coronary atherosclerosis, you will experience heart symptoms more easily. For example, if you lose blood suddenly, as in stomach bleeding or a severe nose bleed, you may feel chest discomfort, since not enough oxygen is getting to the part of your heart served by the narrowed (atherosclerotic) artery. Your symptoms might be mistaken for a heart attack until anemia is identified. When your anemia is corrected, you can expect your heart symptoms to improve.

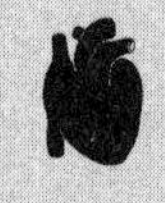

Anemia can be responsible for aggravating heart symptoms.

Hiatus Hernia and Reflux Esophagitis

These two conditions are not the same, though they are often confused with each other. Both can cause chest pain, similar to angina or heart attack symptoms. With both, the pain can be felt in the front of the chest and may radiate to the jaw or arms.

Hiatus Hernia

A hiatus hernia means that the snug opening in the diaphragm, which separates the chest from the abdomen, is too lax. This opening is for the esophagus, which carries swallowed food to your stomach. With a hiatus hernia, part of your stomach can be pinched, causing pain and discomfort similar to that of angina.

Hiatus hernia is usually diagnosed by x-ray of the gastrointestinal tract.

Reflux Esophagitis

Reflux esophagitis, a common cause of heartburn, is an inflammation of the esophagus due to stomach acids rising into the esophagus, where they do not belong. This can occur without a hiatus hernia. It can cause various degrees of chest pain, which can radiate to the arms or jaws, as with angina.

You have valves that prevent stomach acids from regurgitating into your esophagus, but if you have reflux esophagitis, they are faulty.

Peptic Ulcer

Usually found in the stomach or duodenum, peptic ulcers are inflammations of the mucous lining, due to irritation and hyperacidity. Occasionally the pain from these is felt not in the abdomen but in the chest. If you have chest pains due to a peptic ulcer, you may fear it is a heart problem. Diagnostic tests will show the true cause of the pain. Treatment with diet and medication will usually give prompt relief.

Peptic ulcers or gallstones can also produce symptoms similar to angina or a heart attack.

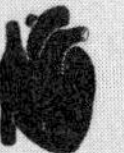

Gallstones or Gallbladder Inflammation

Gallstones can result from crystallization of bile in the gallbladder. You may have gallstones for years without symptoms. Then one night, when they get caught in a narrow passage of the gallbladder, or cause inflammation of that organ, you may wake up with intense pain in the front of your chest or abdomen, causing you to break into a cold sweat and feel nauseated. This is known as gallstone colic.

Although gallstone colic resembles a heart attack, it will not cause the typical test results of a heart attack (e.g. electrocardiographic patterns and blood tests). Gallstones are identified by ultrasonic or x-ray examinations. Until your condition is definitely diagnosed, you should seek emergency help, to be certain that you are not having a heart attack.

Splenic Flexure Syndrome

If you have an irritable (spastic) bowel, you may occasionally feel chest pains that make you fear you have heart trouble. One possible cause for such pain is splenic flexure syndrome. The splenic flexure is a curve of your large bowel near the spleen, on the left-hand side of the abdomen, close to the diaphragm. If gas gets trapped in this section of the bowel, it may cause chest pain that can be confused with heart pains.

Skeletal Factors

Many people have chest or arm pains originating in the neck or chest wall. Spinal cord nerves supplying the chest wall can be pinched by disc disease or arthritis. You can also suffer chest pains due to rheumatic conditions of the chest wall. These are often related to increased stress, which tightens up the chest muscles.

■ SUMMARY

Several conditions unrelated to heart disease can cause symptoms similar to those of a heart attack. If you experience any of these symptoms, see your doctor for a firm diagnosis and treatment.

For Partners and Other Family Members 13

Preventing heart attacks is not just an individual and personal mission. If you are engaged in a heart attack prevention program, your family will be affected in many ways. Your way of life will be altered, and so will that of your family.

■ TALK TO YOUR FAMILY

If you are at risk for a heart attack, you need to tell this to the people you live with, especially your partner. This is important not only for your health, but also for your relationship. Unless there are serious flaws in your relationship, your partner will want to help you with your heart attack prevention program.

You must also share your worries with your family. If you keep your concerns about your health private, for fear of worrying your family, you wrong both yourself and your family. Just talking about what is bothering you can make you feel better, and your family will be better able to help you if they know your concerns.

Talk to your family about your goals. If your family members know what your goals are, they will be able to help you achieve them. Improving your risk factors needs to become a common, family purpose.

Do Not Exaggerate Your Risks

It is important that you do not exaggerate your risks. You must not exploit or appear to exploit the concern of your family. If the members of your family care for you, they will have a natural urge to help.

HOW YOUR FAMILY CAN HELP

To try to change your lifestyle without the help of your family, or members of your household, is virtually impossible. Here are some ways your partner and other family members can help.

- *If you and your partner both smoke, it will be easier for you to quit if your partner also quits and you help each other. If your partner does not quit, you are endangered by the secondhand smoke.* *(See p. 34.)*
- *If you need to lose weight, you must have your family's cooperation. It is impractical to have two diets in the same home. If other members of the family are eating food that you are trying to avoid, your chances of lapsing with your dietary discipline are greater.*
- *If your blood pressure is high, your family will need to be aware of the risk for you, and what needs to be done about it.*
- *Your family can provide invaluable help by encouraging you to exercise, perhaps accompanying you on walks or other activities.*
- *Your partner and other family members must know as much as you do about your heart attack risk factors, and what can be done about them. They should be able to ask questions of your doctor and be encouraged to attend classes, watch videos, or read books on ways to prevent heart attacks.*
- *Family members may want to consider taking a course in cardiopulmonary resuscitation (CPR).*
- *If your partner or another family member is responsible for shopping, he or she needs to become wise in selecting suitable, healthy foods while still having an appealing menu.*

Your family can be your strongest support group, but only if you share your health concerns and goals.

- *When you eat out, you will need cooperation in selecting restaurants where the menu includes heart-healthy items.*
- *Your partner can help you develop your stress-reducing practices.*
- *By listening to your worries and concerns, your partner and other members of your family can help reduce stress, and motivate you to keep up your heart attack prevention program.*

SUMMARY

- *It is important to tell your partner and other members of your family about your heart attack risks, your concerns about yourself, and your goals for heart attack prevention.*
- *This information should be shared without exaggerating your risks.*
- *There are many practical ways that your family can help you reduce your risk factors for a heart attack.*
- *If you and your partner and other family members work together, not only will you be more likely to achieve your goals, but the quality of your relationships will also be improved.*

Reducing your risk factors may involve changes for the whole family, such as quitting smoking.

14 Important New Research

The studies listed below examine the risk effects of differing cholesterol levels, of variations in diets, of supplementation with specific vitamins, and of differing blood levels of certain minerals. Also given are significant results of studies examining the effectiveness of medications like resins, fibric acids, statins, and niacin.

Until very recently, most heart studies used solely men as their subjects. Women were not included partly because they were considered to be at a much lower risk for heart attacks. As outlined in earlier chapters, it is now apparent that a woman's risk factors are different than a man's. The results and recommendations of studies exclusive to men do not necessarily apply to women. Some of the studies noted in the summaries below include women, as their descriptions indicate. Large-scale research on women and heart disease is currently underway.

TYPES OF STUDIES

There are two types of human population studies of diseases: observational studies, and random controlled trials.

In an observational study, people with a certain disease or condition are compared with others who do not have it. For example, patients with high blood cholesterol are studied and compared to people who do not have high cholesterol (the controls).

A random controlled trial compares patients receiving a certain type of treatment to others with the same disease or condition who do not receive the treatment (the controls). The controls receive a placebo that seems identical to the treatment but contains no medication. The patients receiving treatment are chosen at random. Blind trials, where neither the patient nor the doctor knows who is receiving treatment and who is receiving a placebo, are considered especially valid.

Both types of study have been used to find out more about heart disease. Below are the findings of some of the most important studies.

OBSERVATIONAL STUDIES

The Framingham Heart Study (ongoing)

This Massachusetts study has been active for more than 40 years. It began in 1949 with more than 5,000 men and women, aged 30 through 59, who were free from heart disease. Over the years they have been checked and rechecked.

Findings:

- *If you are a man with high cholesterol, you have a greater than average chance of dying at a younger age than men with moderate cholesterol.*
- *If you are a woman, your total cholesterol can be considerably higher before putting you at increased risk.*
- *The ratio of your total cholesterol to HDL cholesterol is a better predictor of heart attack risk than your total cholesterol alone.*

Trans-Fatty Acid Intake Study (1992)
(substudy of ongoing Veterans' Administration Normative Aging Study)

In this Harvard Medical School substudy of 748 healthy

men, the relation between the intake of trans-fatty acids (found in margarines and partially hydrogenated vegetable oils) and blood lipids was assessed.

Findings:

- *Those men who habitually consumed the highest amounts of trans-fatty acids were found to have a 27 percent higher heart attack risk than those who consumed the least.*
- *High trans-fatty acid intake increased total and LDL cholesterol levels, as well as the ratio of total to HDL cholesterol.*

World Health Organization/Monica Project (1991)

This large study involved middle-aged men in 16 European cultures with widely varying heart attack rates. The levels of vitamin E in the men's blood also varied widely.

Findings:

- *The groups with the highest heart attack death rates had the lowest vitamin E levels.*
- *Those with the lowest heart attack death rates had the highest vitamin E levels.*

Kupio (Finland) Ischemic Heart Disease Risk Factor Study (1982, 1992)

Researchers in the 1980s began investigating causes for the unusually high rate of heart attacks in eastern Finland. Subsequent studies of more than 2,000 men with heart disease, between the ages of 42 and 60, and living in eastern Finland, examined levels of minerals in the blood, especially selenium, copper, and iron.

Findings:

- *The mineral selenium was deficient in many heart attack victims.*
- *Excess blood levels of copper and iron were found in many of the observed subjects.*

The Seven Countries Study (1980s)

This 15-year study recorded the clinical histories of 11,579 middle-aged men in Finland, Greece, Italy, Japan, the Netherlands, the United States, and the former Yugoslavia. They were examined every five years for high blood pressure, cholesterol abnormalities, and smoking habits. Their diets were analyzed in detail.

Findings:

- *After 15 years, their death rates were found to correlate with their intake of saturated fats, giving strong evidence that a diet high in saturated fats increases heart attack risk in men.*

The Adventist Health Study (1992) and Subsequent Related Studies

In a study of more than 30,000 Californian Seventh-Day Adventists, people who reported eating nuts more than four times weekly were found to have 50 percent fewer heart attacks. Subsequent reports attributed this beneficial effect to the high level of L-arginine in the protein content of nuts.

L-arginine is the precursor in the body to nitric oxide (NO), considered to be the "endothelial-derived relaxing factor" that has been fascinating scientists in recent years.

In 1994 Stanford University scientists showed that high dietary L-arginine (increasing the intake six-fold) prevented atherosclerosis in rabbits fed a high cholesterol diet.

L-arginine and nitric oxide continue to be the subject of intense interest by both scientific workers and clinicians.

RANDOM CONTROLLED TRIALS

First National Health & Nutrition Examination Survey Follow-up Study (1984)

In this U.S. survey, the diet and health of more than 11,000 men and women between the ages of 25 and 74 were examined. One part of the follow-up study compared vitamin C ingestion with death rates from heart diseases. One group followed their usual diet, which was low in vitamin C (less than 50 mg/day); a second group maintained a diet containing 50 mg or more of vitamin C daily; while a third group ate a high vitamin C diet (more than 50 mg daily), and also took vitamin C supplements averaging several hundred milligrams per day.

Findings:

- *The group that followed a high vitamin C diet and also took supplements greatly reduced their risk of dying from heart disease (by up to 40 percent for men and 20 percent for women).*

Note: A number of studies, including those summarized below, have examined the effects of medications on people at risk for heart attacks. The latest research indicates that for most people lifestyle changes alone are effective, and much safer than treatment with drugs in heart attack prevention. However, if your risk factors indicate you are at high risk, it is advisable to consult with your physician to discuss adding drug treatment to your cholesterol-lowering program.

St. Thomas Atherosclerosis Regression Study (1992)
This British study involved 90 men with coronary artery disease and high cholesterol levels (the average total cholesterol was 280 mg/dL, or 7.23 mmol/L). A control group which continued on a "usual" diet was compared with one group which maintained a strict diet and took the resin cholestyramine, and with another group which stayed on the strict diet alone. The coronary arteries of all the men were restudied after 39 months.

Findings:

- *Men on the rigid diet did as well or better than those who were also given medication, and much better than those on the "usual" diet.*
- *Improved diameter in the arteries could be predicted by improved levels of LDL and HDL cholesterol.*

Familial Atherosclerosis Treatment Study (1990)
This Seattle study was a six-year follow-up of 120 men with a family history of premature heart disease. They were divided into a control group and two treatment groups. One treatment group was given the statin lovastatin and the

resin colestipol, and the other group was given niacin and the resin colestipol.

Findings:

- *Reversal of coronary plaques occurred in a high percentage of men in the treated groups.*
- *There was a highly significant reduction in the rate of subsequent heart attacks and other coronary "events".*
- *Those given lovastatin and colestipol averaged a 48 percent drop in their LDL cholesterol and a 14 percent rise of HDL cholesterol compared to the control group.*
- *Those given niacin and colestipol averaged a 34 percent drop of LDL cholesterol and a 41 percent rise of HDL cholesterol compared to the control group.*

Helsinki Heart Study (1987)

This Finnish study was a five-year follow-up of 4,081 middle-aged men with no evidence of heart disease but with abnormal lipid levels. Half received gemfibrozil, a fibric acid agent to improve blood lipids, and half received a placebo.

Findings:

- *The men receiving gemfibrozil had 26 percent fewer deaths from heart attacks and 37 percent fewer nonfatal heart attacks than the control group.*
- *In the patients whose ratio of total cholesterol to HDL cholesterol fell the most, the number of heart attacks was reduced more markedly.*

Scandinavian Simvastatin Survival Study (4S Study) (1994)

This was a six year study of 4,444 men and women with diseased coronary arteries and blood cholesterol levels of 5.5 millimol per liter or more (210 milligrams per deciliter). They were randomly chosen to receive 20 milligrams or more per day of either a placebo or simvastatin. Both groups had comparable numbers of women and elderly.

Findings:

- *In comparison with the placebo group, patients on simvastatin experienced a 30 percent reduction of all-cause mortality; 42 per-*

cent reduction of mortality from coronary disease and a 34 percent reduction in major nonfatal coronary events such as heart attacks, need for by-pass grafts or angioplasty.

- *Patients on simvastatin experienced dramatic improvement in their lipid levels.*
- *Those given simvastatin also had very few problems with side-effects (drop-outs in treatment group, 10 percent; from placebo group; 13 percent).*

SUMMARY

To date, heart disease studies have shown that:

- *If you are a man, you have a greater chance of dying at a younger age if your cholesterol is high.*
- *If you are a woman, high total cholesterol appears not to put you at increased risk for a heart attack. (However, if your total cholesterol level is over 265 mg/dL, or 6.85 mmol/L, you should have a careful assessment of your risk for heart disease.)*
- *The ratio of total cholesterol to HDL cholesterol is an important risk factor for either sex.*
- *The antioxidant vitamins C and E are linked to a lower death rate from heart disease.*
- *The antioxidant mineral selenium is linked with lower copper and iron levels in the blood, and a lower heart attack rate.*
- *Diets high in saturated fats are linked with a higher death rate from heart attacks.*
- *Foods rich in the amino acid L-arginine (such as nuts, seeds, and legumes) may be important for heart attack prevention.*
- *Coronary atherosclerosis can often be reversed when LDL and HDL cholesterol levels are sufficiently improved by strict attention to diet and other lifestyle changes.*
- *If you have coronary disease, radical improvement of your cholesterol levels dramatically lowers your risk of heart attack and other coronary events.*
- *Coronary disease patients with cholesterol levels 210 (5.5) or more, if treated with sufficient simvastatin to dramatically improve their cholesterol levels, can significantly reduce their risk of further coronary heart complications with a low risk of side effects.*

Appendices: Guides for a Heart-Healthy Diet

A: FAT CALORIES & SATURATED FAT CALORIES IN COMMON FOODS

The percentages of fat calories and saturated fat calories are derived from the total calories in a food. Do not confuse the result with the percentage of fat *weight* of a food. For example, while milk may contain 2 percent fat by weight, it contains 37 percent fat calories, of which 22 percent are saturated fat calories.

If you are at risk for heart attacks and your cholesterol needs to be reduced, keep fat calories to less than 30 percent and saturated fat calories to less than 10 percent of total calories consumed. It is saturated fat that drives up your cholesterol levels, especially the LDL (bad) cholesterol.

Not included in the table are foods with very low fat calories. Don't forget that the food items listed below have less than 10 percent fat calories and negligible amounts of saturated fat. These are the foods you can exploit to reduce your cholesterol levels.

- *Legumes: beans, peas, lentils*
- *Tubers: potatoes, carrots, turnips*
- *Vegetables and fruits: all, except avocados and olives*
- *Whole grain cereals*
- *Rice, flour, pasta*

The following data were calculated from values of fat and calories from selected food items in *The Handbook of the Nutritional Value of Foods in Common Units*, Catherine F. Adams, for the United States Department of Agriculture (New York: Dover Publications, 1986), and *Food Values: Cholesterol and Fats*, Leah Wallach (New York: Harper and Row, 1989). Percent fat values were determined by multiplying the grams of fat (total fat and saturated fat respectively) by nine to determine the fat calories, then calculating the quotient of the total calories/fat (or saturated fat) calories.

PERCENTAGE OF FAT CALORIES AND SATURATED FAT CALORIES IN COMMON FOODS

Note: The percentages of fat and saturated fat calories for the meat items listed below are for meats prepared using lean cooking methods, such as braising, broiling, or roasting.

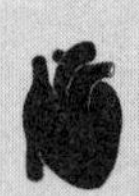

Keep fat calories under 30% and saturated fat calories under 10% of your total calorie intake.

The percentages for seafoods refer to the raw seafood, except as marked. When seafoods are prepared using lean cooking methods, such as baking, broiling, microwaving, or steaming, the percentages will be very close to those for the raw food.

The fat percentages given in the left-hand column refers to the percentage of fat contained in a food by *weight,* rather than by calories.

	% Fat Calories	% Saturated Fat Calories
Beef		
Boneless chuck and chuck cuts		
18% fat (for stew)	69	33
15% fat	60	29

	% Fat Calories	% Saturated Fat Calories
Chuck rib steak or roast		
30% fat	80	39
Club steak		
42% fat	80	39
trimmed of separable fat	48	23
Porterhouse steak		
43% fat	82	39
trimmed of separable fat	42	20
Round steak		
19% fat	53	26
trimmed of separable fat	29	14
Sirloin, loin end		
34% fat	74	36
trimmed of separable fat	33	16
T-bone steak		
44% fat	82	39
trimmed of separable fat	42	20
Rib roast		
36% fat	80	39
trimmed of separable fat	50	24
Rump roast		
25% fat	71	34
trimmed of separable fat	40	19
Ground beef		
10% fat	46	22
20% fat	64	31
Pork		
Roast, loin		
20% fat	71	25
trimmed of separable fat	50	18
Shoulder		
26% fat	73	31

	% Fat Calories	% Saturated Fat Calories
Spare ribs		
lean, but including fat	79	29
Ham		
16% fat	69	25
light, lean, but including fat	70	25
lean only	54	19
Bacon		
side	79	25
Canadian	60	22
Lamb		
Leg, without bone		
17% fat	66	37
trimmed of separable fat	34	19
Loin chops		
34% fat	74	42
trimmed of separable fat	36	20
Shoulder		
26% fat	72	41
trimmed of separable fat	44	25
Poultry		
Turkey (roasted)		
without skin: dark meat	36	11
without skin: light meat	18	5
with skin	56	16
Chicken (roasted)		
without skin: dark meat	32	10
without skin: light meat	18	6
with skin	52	17

	% Fat Calories	% Saturated Fat Calories
Fish		
Cod, Atlantic or Pacific (raw)	13	—
Flounder (raw)	11	—
Haddock (raw)	12	—
Halibut, Atlantic or Pacific (raw)	19	—
Herring, Atlantic (raw)	54	13
Herring, Greenland (raw)	68	11
Mackerel, Atlantic (raw)	62	15
Perch, ocean (raw)	11	—
Pike, northern (raw)	12	—
Salmon, Atlantic (raw)	37	7
Salmon, chinook (canned)	60	18
Salmon, chum (raw)	26	9
Salmon, coho (raw)	36	7
Salmon, pink (raw)	27	—
canned (solids & liquid)	37	7
Salmon, sockeye (raw)	44	6
Sardines, Atlantic (canned in oil)	54	—
Snapper (raw)	10	—
Swordfish (raw)	26	9
Trout, rainbow (raw)	27	9
Tuna, bluefin (raw)	30	7
canned in oil	37	10
Shellfish		
Clams (raw)	14	—
breaded and fried	50	12
Crab, white or king (raw)	14	—
Crab, Dungeness (raw)	13	—
Crayfish, mixed species (raw)	9	—
Lobster, northern (raw)	12	—

	% Fat Calories	% Saturated Fat Calories
Mussels, blue (raw)	25	—
Oysters, eastern (raw)	31	15
breaded and fried	59	16
Oysters, Pacific (raw)	26	—
Scallops (raw)	12	—
breaded and fried	40	13
Shrimp, mixed species (raw)	10	1
breaded and fried	44	9
Pasta		
Macaroni (enriched)	5	—
Spaghetti (enriched)	3	—
Dairy Products		
Milk		
whole	48	31
2%	37	22
1%	27	14
skim	5	3
evaporated unsweetened		
whole	50	31
skim	4	1
sweetened condensed	25	6
Buttermilk (fresh)	18	12
dried	14	8
Cream		
half-and-half (11.7% fat)	79	43
light or coffee (20.6% fat)	87	48
heavy or whipping (37.6% fat)	95	53
Sour cream	87	55
Yogurt, plain, with added milk solids		
made with low-fat milk	25	14
made with whole milk	45	31

	% Fat Calories	% Saturated Fat Calories
Ice cream, regular (11% fat)	48	30
Sherbet (about 2% fat)	13	8
Butter	100	55
Margarine		
regular, hard	100	19
regular, soft and whipped	100	19

Note: *Avoid hydrogenated fats. Try to find spreads that are nonhydrogenated. The trans-fatty acids resulting from this process cause your* LDL *cholesterol to rise while your hdl cholesterol declines. In addition, most margarines have chemical additives.*

Cheese		
Blue or Roquefort	75	41
Camembert	74	41
Cheddar, domestic	73	40
Limburger	73	40
Mozzarella		
whole milk	70	44
partly skimmed milk	56	35
Parmesan	72	35
Pasteurized processed		
American	73	40
Swiss	66	43
Swiss, domestic	68	37
Cottage cheese		
Dry curd, with creaming mixture (4.2% milk fat)	36	20
Cream cheese	91	50

Legumes		
Chickpeas (garbanzos)	12	1
Kidney beans, red	4	—
Lima beans	4	—

	% Fat Calories	% Saturated Fat Calories
Navy beans	4	—
Soybeans	40	6
Tofu	38	8

B: COMMON FOODS COMPARED BY SATURATED FAT CONTENT

Choose	Avoid
Skim milk, 1% milk	Whole milk, 2% milk
Soy milk	Regular evaporated milk, condensed cream, half-and-half, all imitation dairy products
Skim-milk or low-fat cheeses	Whole-milk or all-natural (unprocessed) cheeses, such as camembert, cheddar, swiss, blue
Low-fat yogurt	Sour cream
Ice milk, frozen low-fat yogurt	Ice cream
Naturally processed oils, nonhydrogenated spreads	Hard margarines and other hydrogenated spreads
Foods cooked by microwave, broiling, boiling, poaching	Foods fried, deep-fried, roasted
Foods cooked with olive, canola, or other unsaturated vegetable oil	Foods cooked with lard or bacon grease
Lean beef or pork, skinless turkey or chicken, tofu	Prepared meats: sausages, wieners, sandwich meats; organ meats, roasts, fatty steaks, spare ribs

Choose	Avoid
Fish: broiled, steamed, poached	Fish: deep-fried, fried
Baked or boiled potatoes	French fries, potato chips, fried potatoes
All vegetables	Vegetables in butter, cream, or cheese sauces
Fruits	Fruit pies

■ C: OMEGA 3 CONTENT OF FISH

	Approximate Amount (in mg) in 3.5 Ounces (100g)
Sardines	5,000
Pacific salmon (chinook)	3,000
Atlantic mackerel	2,500
Pink salmon	1,900
Atlantic herring	1,600
Bluefish	1,400
Atlantic salmon	1,200
Rainbow trout	1,000
Alaska king crab	600
Tuna	500
Atlantic cod	300
Shrimp	300
Flounder or haddock	200
Swordfish	200

■ D: VITAMINS & MINERALS IMPORTANT FOR HEART ATTACK PREVENTION

Vitamins & Minerals: Benefits	Food Sources	Suggested Daily Supplement
Beta carotene (pro-vitamin A): Antioxidant.	Carrots, yams	25,000 IU (15mg)
Vitamin B_1 (thiamine): Aids methionine metabolism; may help resist athero-sclerosis.	Cereals, grains, wheat germ, brewers' yeast	5mg
Vitamin B_3 (niacin): Aids lipid levels at high doses.	Liver, bran, legumes, yeast	1.5–3g
Vitamin B_6 (pyridoxine): Raises hdl in some cases.	Cereals, grains, meats	2–5mg
Vitamin B_{12} (cyanocobalamin): Aids methionine metabolism; may help resist atherosclerosis.	Liver	3mcg
Vitamin C (ascorbic acid): Antioxidant.	Fresh fruits, vegetables	1g

Vitamins & Minerals: Benefits	Food Sources	Suggested Daily Supplement
Vitamin E (alpha tocopheral): Antioxidant.	Cereals, grains	800 IU
Chromium: Supplements may improve cholesterol levels and glucose metabolism.	Grains, whole grain cereals, brewer's yeast	25mcg
Magnesium: Improves heart blood flow and lipids; protects against sudden death.	Beans, nuts, leafy vegetables, hard water	100–500mg
Selenium: Antioxidant; adds to benefit of vitamin E.	Legumes, seafood, grains, dairy products, tomatoes, cabbage	25mcg
Zinc: Important for many enzyme reactions in the body. Use with caution; don't exceed suggested amount.	Meat, eggs, liver, seafood, wheat germ	15–25mg

■ E: FOODS RICH IN L.ARGININE

More or less than 1,000 milligrams per serving

Meats*	Beef Pork Veal Lamb Poultry
Fish	Most species, including Salmon, Tuna, Cod, Halibut, etc.
Shell Fish	Shrimp (3 ounces)
Legumes	Red, Navy, Lima Beans** Lentils Chik Peas
Nuts	Pine Nuts Soybean Nuts (dry roasted) Walnuts (black, dried)
Seeds	Pumpkin Seeds Squash Seeds

** Servings of 3½ ounces generally supply considerably more than 1000 milligrams of L-arginine.*
*** This group of beans contains slightly less than 1000 milligrams per cup.*

Glossary of Medical Terms

ACE inhibitors: See *Angiotensin converting enzyme inhibitors*

Acetylsalicylic acid (ASA): The chemical term for aspirin.

Aerobic exercise: Exercise (such as running or swimming) to improve respiration and circulation, by increasing oxygen consumption.

Amino acids: Nitrogen-containing compounds which are the building blocks of protein.

Anemia: A deficiency of hemoglobin in the blood. See also *Hemoglobin.*

Aneurysm: A bulge in an artery wall, often where the wall has been weakened by atherosclerosis. See also *Atherosclerosis.*

Angina (angina pectoris): Pain or discomfort, usually in the front of the chest, due to insufficient blood flow to the heart muscle.

Angiogram: An x-ray of the inner cavity (lumen) of an artery, taken by injecting a dye that is opaque to the x-rays.

Angioplasty: Widening an artery to improve its ability to carry blood by (1) inflating a tube within the artery; (2) using laser rays to destroy the obstructing portion of the artery; or (3) inserting a specialized instrument inside the artery, to chip away the obstructing plaque.

Angiotensin converting enzyme (ACE) inhibitors: Medicinal agents used to treat high blood pressure and congestive heart failure.

Antioxidant: A substance, such as vitamin C, that inhibits oxidation. See also *Oxidation.*

Aorta: The major artery delivering blood from the heart to the body by means of its various branches.

Arcus senilis: Gray lines in the form of an arc, in the iris of the eyes.

ASA: See *Acetylsalicylic acid*

Asthma: A condition associated with labored breathing, chest constriction, and coughing due to congested bronchial tubes. Often caused by allergies.

Atherosclerosis: A common degenerative disease of the arteries, caused by a build-up of plaque, and developing over a period of years. The main cause of blocked arteries, and a common cause of heart attacks.

Atypical chest pain: Chest pain which is not typical of angina pectoris.

Beta blockers (beta adrenergic blockers): Medications that block certain sympathetic nerves to the heart and arteries (and other organs), causing a slower heart beat and lower blood pressure.

Beta carotene: One of the several red or orange pigments in plants, or the fat of plant-eating animals, that can be converted to vitamin A after ingestion. It has important antioxidant effects. Also called pro-vitamin A.

Blinded trial: An experiment, designed to eliminate bias, on a number of subjects to test the value of a treatment. The trial may be *single blinded*, where the subjects do not know whether they are receiving a medication or a placebo; or *double blinded*, where neither the subjects nor the medical supervisors know which person is receiving the medication. See also *Placebo; Random controlled trial.*

Blood platelets: Small corpuscles in the bloodstream responsible for sealing wounds. In damaged arteries, blood platelets can cause unwanted blood clots. See also *Coronary thrombosis.*

Bronchial asthma: An illness causing shortness of breath and heavy discomfort in the chest due to narrowing of the bronchial tubes.

Bruit: A sound resulting from blood flowing over a narrowed artery, heard with a stethoscope.

Burnout syndrome: A chronic state of unwellness accompanied by fatigue, poor concentration, and anxiety. Due to chronic, or severe, emotional stress.

Calcium score: A measurement of the density and extensiveness of calcium deposits in the coronary arteries as shown by ultrafast computerized x-rays of the coronary arteries.

Carbon monoxide: A poisonous gas inhaled with cigarette smoke.

Cardiac catheter: A specialized hollow tube designed to enter the inside of the heart, by passing into and through an accessible artery, usually in the groin.

Cardiomyopathy: A disease of the heart muscle, usually not associated with coronary artery disease.

Cardiopulmonary resuscitation (CPR): An emergency and temporary procedure on a person who has collapsed from cardiac arrest, to prevent the brain suffering from lack of oxygen. Mouth-to-mouth blowing of air into the lungs is combined with rhythmic pressure of the chest wall, over the heart.

Chelation therapy: Treatments aimed at reducing certain heavy metal deposits in the body, such as calcium, by administering a chelation agent (EDTA), which binds with the metal.

Cholesterol: A fatty substance necessary for life and health, found in our blood and tissues. It is transported in the blood by lipoprotein. Abnormal arterial build-up of cholesterol is an important component of cholesterol plaque. See also *High density lipoprotein cholesterol; Low density lipoprotein cholesterol; Plaque.*

Chronic obstructive lung disease (emphysema): A disease associated with difficulty breathing due to bronchial narrowing, or loss of lung elasticity (commonly due to cigarette smoking).

Chronic stable angina: Predictable angina, usually occurring with a certain level of exercise and relieved promptly with resting.

Congestive heart failure: The result of weakness of the pumping action of the heart, causing congestion of various organs, including the lungs and liver.

Coronary angiography: The procedure of taking angiograms of the coronary arteries.

Coronary artery: The arteries responsible for transporting and distributing blood to the heart muscle.

Coronary artery bypass graft: Surgically bypassing a narrowed coronary artery, allowing blood to flow freely to the heart muscle. An artery from within the chest cavity (the internal mammary artery), or a leg vein, is grafted from the aorta to a coronary artery past the obstructed area.

Coronary artery disease: A common term for atherosclerosis of the coronary arteries.

Coronary artery plaque: A thickened area of the inner lining of a coronary artery, due to atherosclerosis. See also *Atherosclerosis;Cholesterol.*

Coronary atherosclerosis: Atherosclerosis of the coronary arteries. See also *Atherosclerosis.*

Coronary thrombosis: An acute closure of a coronary artery due to a blood clot (thrombus), superimposed on atherosclerosis, resulting in a heart attack, myocardial infarct, or sudden cardiac death. See also *Atherosclerosis;Myocardial infarct.*

CPR: See *Cardiopulmonary resuscitation*

Deciliter (dL): one tenth of a liter.

Diastolic blood pressure: The blood pressure in the arteries when the heart is in the resting phase. See also *Systolic blood pressure.*

Dipyridamole: A pharmaceutical substance that dilates the outer arteries of the heart, causing the blood to shunt away from the interior muscles. Simulates the effects of exercise. See also *Mibi scan.*

Diuretic: A pharmaceutical or natural substance that stimulates the production of urine by the kidneys.

Dobutamine: A pharmaceutical agent that causes the heart rate and blood pressure to rise, simulating the effects of exercise.

Dobutamine stress test: For those unable to exercise, this test checks whether suspected coronary atherosclerosis impedes blood flow in the heart by simulating the effects of exercise. See also *Mibi; Thallium scan.*

Echocardiogram: A test using ultrasound waves to reflect the dimensions of the heart, both in its contracting and relaxing phase.

Eicosapentoic acid (EPA): A polyunsaturated fatty acid, belonging to the omega 3 family, necessary to the human body, found primarily in fish oil.

Electrocardiogram (EKG,ECG): Shows the normal or abnormal waveforms from the electrical activity during the heart's contraction and relaxation.

Emphysema: See *Chronic obstructive lung disease*

EPA: See *Eicosapentoic acid*

Estrogens: Pre-menopausal hormones secreted from the ovaries, and commercially available in pills, injectables, and skin patches.

False positive exercise test: An exercise test that gives the same readings as those seen in coronary atherosclerosis, but where this condition is later shown not to be present.

Familial hypercholesterolemia: High blood cholesterol levels in a person with a family history of premature deaths, and close relatives who have had high blood cholesterol levels.

Fibric acid agents: Pharmaceuticals that are used to lower low density lipoprotein (LDL) cholesterol and triglycerides, and raise high density lipoprotein (HDL) cholesterol.

Fibrous cap: The layer of fibrous tissue on the inner (bloodstream) side of an atherosclerotic plaque.

Gamma camera: A camera designed to detect radioactivity.

Genetic: Inherited, via the genes.

Hard water: Water containing a high content of minerals, especially calcium and magnesium.

HDL: See *High density lipoprotein*

Heart attack: A sudden illness due to a heart disturbance, usually an acute closure of a coronary artery. See also *Coronary thrombosis; Myocardial infarct.*

Hemoglobin: The red pigment of blood cells, which contains iron and carries oxygen to the body's tissues.

High density lipoprotein (HDL): The more densely packed blood lipoproteins, in contrast to similar loosely packed molecules.

High density lipoprotein (HDL) cholesterol: The "good" cholesterol carried by HDL molecules, which combats atherosclerosis. See also *Low density lipoprotein cholesterol.*

Hydrogenated fats: Vegetable fats that are ordinarily liquid and unsaturated, but have been altered by manufacturers to be more solid (and more saturated), by forcing hydrogen ions onto their molecules. Hydrogenated and saturated fats are primary causes of high blood levels of low density lipoprotein (LDL) cholesterol. See also *Saturated fats.*

Hypertrophy: Increased size of muscular tissue or an organ, usually due to extra work demands.

Hypoglycemia: Low blood sugar.

Insulin: A natural hormone secreted by the pancreas, which affects the metabolism of the body in several ways, including lowering blood sugar.

International units (IU): Units to measure the strength of biological activity of such substances as vitamins, according to international standards. Also refers to *International system of units*, an internationally accepted system of measurement based on metric units of weight.

Irritable bowel: An affliction that usually causes abdominal pain or discomfort, and irregular bowel function.

Ischemia: Insufficient oxygen in tissues, which may be due to atherosclerosis of their feeder arteries.

L-arginine: One of the many amino acids assembled to form a protein molecule.

LDL: See *Low density lipoprotein*

Left ventricular hypertrophy: Hypertrophy of the muscles of the heart's left ventricle.

Lipids: Fats, especially in the bloodstream, including cholesterol and triglycerides.

Lipoproteins: Complex molecules made of fat and protein which transport cholesterol in the bloodstream.

Low density lipoproteins (LDL): Lipoproteins that, when compacted, are loosely packed.

Low density lipoprotein (LDL) *cholesterol:* The "bad" cholesterol carried by LDL molecules, which is linked with atherosclerosis. See also *High density lipoprotein cholesterol.*

Meta-analysis: An analysis of several studies with enough common qualities that the results of the meta-analysis can add strength to the conclusions of the individual studies.

Metabolism: The continuous process of building up and tearing down vital aspects of body cells.

Methionine: An essential amino acid present in many food proteins. Imbalances have been implicated in some cases of premature coronary disease.

Mibi scan: Detects coronary atherosclerosis by injecting radioactive sestamibi into veins. Compares patterns of the radioactive material in the heart muscle before and after exercise, or the injection of dipyridamole.

Milligrams (mg): one thousandth of a gram.

Millimoles (mmol): one thousandth of a gram molecule.

Monounsaturated fats: Fatty acids whose molecular chain has just one unsaturated bond (not occupied by a hydrogen atom). See also *Polyunsaturated fats;Saturated fats.*

Myocardial infarct (or infarction): Death of a portion of the heart muscle deprived of its blood supply, usually as a result of a coronary thrombosis.

Myocardial ischemia: Insufficient oxygen in heart tissues.

Near-maximal exercise test: A test in which a patient, while connected to an electrocardiogram, exercises sufficiently to cause the heart rate to reach its estimated highest rate.

Niacin: Vitamin B_3, also known as nicotinic acid. A naturally occurring substance, which in large doses improves cholesterol and triglyceride levels.

Nicotine: A poisonous substance present in tobacco smoke.

Nonspecific ST segment depression: Abnormal downward shift of the *ST segment* of the electrocardiogram waveform. See also *st* segment.

Omega 3 fatty acids: Polyunsaturated fatty acids with the end unsaturated bond on the third from last carbon atom. See also *Eicosapentoic acid;Polyunsaturated fats.*

Omega 6 fatty acids: Polyunsaturated fatty acids with the end unsaturated bond on the sixth from the last carbon atom. See also *Polyunsaturated fats.*

Ophthalmoscope: Instrument with a special light to view the retina of the eye.

Oxidation: The combination of a substance with oxygen. When LDL cholesterol becomes oxidized, its nature changes, causing it to kindle the process of atherosclerosis.

Pectin: A water-soluble fiber present in certain plant foods.

Pericarditis: Inflammation of the outer lining of the heart, and the surface of the cavity surrounding the heart.

Peroxidation: The chemical process which forms a molecule containing abundant oxygen (for example hydrogen peroxide).

Placebo: A substance containing no medication, used as a control in experiments. See also *Blinded trial;Random controlled trial.*

Plaque: A thickened area on the inner lining of an artery, composed of cholesterol, and fibrous and muscle tissues. See also *Atherosclerosis;Cholesterol.*

Polymer: A chemical compound, made of up to millions of repeated joined units, each one a relatively simple molecule.

Polyunsaturated fats: Fatty acids with more than one unsaturated bond (not occupied by a hydrogen atom) along the chain of carbon atoms. See also *Monounsaturated fats:Saturated fats.*

Post-traumatic stress disorder: See *Burnout syndrome*

Premature heart attack: Heart attack in someone before the age of 55.

Premature ventricular contraction (PVC): A heartbeat a fraction of a second early in the cadence of the normal heart rhythm.

Progesterone: A female hormone secreted by the ovaries, but employed in certain pharmaceuticals, including birth control pills.

Psychological defences: A person's habitual defences against disturbing emotions.

PVC: See *Premature ventricular contraction*

Radionuclide: A nuclide (an atom with special numbers of protons, neutrons, and energy in its nucleus) with radioactive qualities.

Random controlled trial: An experimental study on a number of subjects to test the value of a treatment. Subjects are chosen to receive either the treatment or a placebo (nontreatment) according to "the luck of the draw," to avoid human bias. See also *Blinded trial;Placebo.*

Ratio of total cholesterol/HDL cholesterol: A proven risk indicator for heart attacks, calculated by dividing the total cholesterol by the high density lipoprotein (HDL) cholesterol. For example, a total cholesterol of 300 divided by HDL cholesterol of 75 gives a ratio of 4 to 1, typically written as 4.

Risk factor: An indicator showing a person's increased risk for a disease, such as a heart attack.

Saturated fats: Fatty acids in which the chains of carbon atoms are completely occupied by their quota of hydrogen atoms, and thus saturated. See also *Hydrogenated fats; Mono-unsaturated fats; Polyunsaturated fats.*

Silent exertional ischemia: Ischemia (insufficient oxygen in tissues) affecting a part of the heart muscle during exertion, without showing any symptoms.

Soft water: Water that has a low content of minerals, such as calcium and magnesium.

Stable angina: Angina pectoris, usually experienced with exertion, but in a predictable way, due to that person's past experience with it. See also *Angina; Unstable angina.*

Statin: A family of pharmaceuticals used to improve levels of blood lipids (cholesterol and triglycerides).

Stress test: A test that monitors the way the heart responds to such stress as exertion.

ST segment: A wave on an electrocardiographic pattern, which helps to show the effects of ischemia.

ST segment depression: A downward shift of the ST segment, as occurs with ischemia.

ST segment shift: A change in the alignment of the ST segment with other electrocardiographic pattern waves, often revealing ischemia.

Systemic: Referring to internal body processes. A medication may be absorbed into the blood, where it is distributed systemically. In contrast, it may not be absorbed, but have a more localized effect.

Systolic blood pressure: The blood pressure measured when the heart is contracting, as opposed to relaxing. See also *Diastolic blood pressure.*

Technitium: A metallic element derived from molybdenum, used for medical testing.

Thallium scan: Similar to a mibi scan, but using radioactive thallium. See *Mibi scan.*

Tomography: A special x-ray technique to focus on various (usually) horizontal planes of body tissues, to provide more detail.

Trans-fatty acids: Naturally occurring fatty acids are converted to trans-fatty acids when vegetable oils are hydrogenated. These raise LDL cholesterol levels and promote atherosclerosis. See also *Atherosclerosis; Hydrogenated fats; Low density lipoprotein cholesterol.*

Triglyceride: A lipid in the blood which, when in excess, is a heart attack risk factor.

Ultrafast computerized tomography: A specialized x-ray showing views of an organ in thin layers and at high speed, like "freezing" views of the beating heart.

Ultrasound: Waves that can be emitted from specialized equipment. They cast shadows useful for reflecting anatomical structures, such as heart valves.

Unsaturated fats: Fatty acids in which the chains of carbon atoms are not completely occupied by hydrogen atoms, and are thus unsaturated. See also *Monounsaturated fats;Polyunsaturated fats;Saturated fats.*

Unstable angina: Angina which is experienced unpredictably, often when at rest. See also *Angina;Stable angina.*

Uric acid: A chemical from the metabolism of protein that can be measured in the blood. Excesses can cause gout or kidney stones.

Valvular heart disease (*VHD*): Heart disease as a result of one or more faulty heart valves.

Vaso-vagal syncope: Fainting from a common cause, often from standing for long periods, or from unpleasant sights or smells.

Xanthomata: Yellowish cholesterol deposits, smaller than a grain of rice, seen especially in the skin around the eyes, usually in people with high blood cholesterol.

Suggested Readings

Cholesterol and Coronary Heart Disease:The Great Debate, edited by Phil Gold, md, Steven Grover, md, and Daniel A.K. Roncari, md. Parthenon, Park Ridge, NJ, 1992. Read this book, or parts of it, for an up-to-date series of chapters from worldwide researchers. Some question what was once the medically accepted role of cholesterol in heart disease.

Culture,Health and Illness, Cecil G. Helman. Butterworth, London, 1990. An insight into the symbolic significance of heart trouble, and how society reacts to it.

Detox, Phyllis Saifer, md and Merla Zellerbach. Jeremy P. Tarcher, Los Angeles, 1984. A supportive program for freeing your body from chemical pollutants (at home and at work), junk food additives, sugar, nicotine, drugs, alcohol, and more. Procedures to help break lifelong habits, emphasizing safe and sensible techniques for minimizing physical and psychological effects of withdrawal. A list of detoxification centers is included.

The Female Heart: The Truth about Women and Coronary Heart Disease, Marianne J. Legato, md and Carol Colman. Prentice Hall, New York, 1991. For decades, women have been neglected in studies of coronary artery disease. This book gives the results of recent studies.

Food Values: Cholesterol and Fats, Leah Wallach. Harper and Row, New York, 1989. This handy little book provides useful data on thousands of food items.

Food Values of Portions Commonly Used, 15th ed., Jean A.T. Pennington. Harper Perennial, New York, 1989. This very handy book provides information not only on calories, cholesterol, and fat, but also on salt, sugar, and vitamins.

Healing Your Heart, Henry Hellerstein, md and Paul Perry. Simon and Schuster, New York, 1990. If you have coronary artery disease, this book discusses reversing the obstructions in your arteries via lifestyle changes. Also provides interesting recipes.

Heart to Heart: A Guide to the Psychological Aspect of Heart Disease, Herbert N. Budnick with Scott Robert Hays. Health Press, Santa Fe, 1990. A useful resource on how to overcome the emotional and psychological pitfalls that can affect a heart patient and his or her family.

Learning to Live Well with Diabetes, Marion J. Franz, Donnel D. Etzwiler, md, Judy Ostrom Joynes, Priscilla M. Hollander, md. dci Publishing, Minneapolis, 1991. A comprehensive book for the lay person.

A Little Relaxation, Saul Miller, md. Hartley & Marks, Point Roberts, WA, 1991. A short, easy-reading book showing step by step how busy people can help heal themselves with relaxation techniques.

Living with Angina: A Cardiologist's Guide to Causes, Symptoms, Diagnosis, Treatment, The Doctor-Patient Relationship, and How to Lead a Normal and Productive Life, James A. Pantano, md. Harper and Row, New York, 1990. The title is self-explanatory. If you suffer from angina, this is a good resource.

The Oats, Beans, Peas, Barley Cookbook, 2nd ed., Edith Young Cottrell. Woodbridge Press, Santa Barbara, 1992. These food items are especially healthful for your heart. Emphasizes simplicity, variety (450 recipes), and has many practical features.

Preventive Cardiology, Dennis M. Davidson, md. Williams and Wilkins, Baltimore, 1991. Quite easy to read. Comprehensive, with chapters on epidemiology, risk indicators, and prevention of heart attacks and sudden cardiac death. The author is director of the Preventive Cardiology Clinic at Stanford University.

Reversing Heart Disease, Julian Whitaker, md. Warner Books, New

York, 1985. Discusses the danger of coronary artery disease if you live in North America, and the prevalence of bypass surgery. Emphasizes prevention and reversing heart disease. Includes recipes.

Seafoods and Fish Oils in Human Health and Disease, John E. Kinsella, md. Marcel Dekker, New York, 1987. Presents valuable information from animal studies with applications to human health.

Take Heart! Terence Kavanaugh, md. Key Porter, Toronto, 1992. Covers causes, risk factors, treatment, and rehabilitation for heart patients in detail. Emphasizes the value of exercise.

Taking Control of Your Blood Pressure: Steps to a Healthier Lifestyle, Lorna Milkovitch, Beverly Whitmore, and Peter Henderson. The Foothills Provincial General Hospital and Script: The Writers Group, Calgary, AB, 1991. Written with friendly language and appealing graphics. Helpful for those with high blood pressure.

A Textbook on EDTA Chelation Therapy, edited by Elmer M. Cranton (foreword by Linus Pauling). Human Sciences Press Inc., New York, 1989. A comprehensive and informative book on the theoretical and scientific basis of chelation therapy, with a chapter on artery disease and a bibliography of studies.

Vitamin Intake and Health: A Scientific Review, Suzanne Gaby, Adrienne Bendich, Vishwa Singh, and Lawrence J. Machlin. Marcel Dekker, New York, 1991. A useful review of scientific vitamin research, including valuable antioxidants.

Index

INDEX

NOTES

NOTES

NOTES

NOTES

NOTES